Our Parkinson's Disease Instruction Manual

How to have a good life while living with Parkinson's disease

By Edmund H. Smith, Jr.
and Jane Masterson

Version 1.0

Disclaimer and Terms of Use Agreement

The publisher and the authors are providing this book and its contents on an "as is" basis and make no representations or warranties of any kind with respect to this book or its contents. The publisher and the authors deny all such representations and warranties, including but not limited to warranties of healthcare for a particular purpose. In addition, the publisher and the author assume no responsibility for errors, inaccuracies, omissions, or any other inconsistencies herein.

The content of this book is for informational purposes only and is not intended to diagnose, treat, cure, or prevent any condition or disease. You must understand that this book is not intended as a substitute for consultation with a licensed practitioner. Please consult with your own physician or healthcare specialist regarding the suggestions and recommendations made in this book. The use of this book implies your acceptance of this disclaimer. Therefore, if you wish to apply ideas contained within this book, you are taking full responsibility for your actions.

The publisher and the author make no guarantees concerning the level of success you may experience by following the advice and strategies contained in this book, and you accept the risk that results may differ for every individual. The testimonials and examples provided in this book may show exceptional results, which may not apply to the average reader, and are not intended to represent or guarantee that you will achieve the same or similar results.

The authors and publishers do not warrant the performance, effectiveness or applicability of any sites listed or linked in this book.

Table of Contents

INTRODUCTION

Jane Masterson (Jane), the person with Parkinson's (PWP), and Edmund H. Smith Jr. (Ed) have coexisted with Parkinson's for many years. Together, they have learned how to live a good life regardless of the presence of the disease.

Five years ago, they were asked by their support group to speak about what they had learned about coping with the challenges of everyday life.

Ed and Jane's one-hour presentation, "Ideas for Living Well with Parkinson's Disease," proved an instant success. They have been frequent speakers at support groups on the west coast of Florida, eastern Tennessee, and on cruise ships, to audiences of just a few to well over one hundred.

Here are some of the comments from attendees:

"Best Parkinson's presentation we have ever attended."

"I wish I had attended your presentation soon after I was diagnosed."

"We have adopted many of the things you mentioned."

"Can you provide us a written copy of your presentation?"

"You should write a book so more people can benefit from what you have learned."

Recently, after a presentation, a woman came up to Ed with tears in her eyes, embraced him, and thanked him and Jane for giving hope to her and her husband. They had been devastated by his recent Parkinson's diagnosis, but, as result of the presentation, now understood that such a diagnosis does not mean that they will not experience an enjoyable and rewarding life. One simply needs to adapt, and benefit from the experiences of others.

That did it for Jane and Ed. They decided to write an autobiography, with the hope that they might make a positive impact in the lives of others by sharing what they have learned during their 25-year journey, with a constant companion, Parkinson's disease.

Ed and Jane welcome comments from their readers. Email them at the follow address:

parkinson.educators@gmail.com

Jane decided that Ed should write most of our book while she offered advice and supervision. So, come with us on our journey, with Ed at the keyboard!

CHAPTER 1 – Parkinson's and Us

Our story begins in early 1997, when Jane's bank rejected a check she had written, claiming the signature did not match the one on file. Her handwriting had become unreadable. She had also noticed that when she walked, her dominant arm did not swing, but instead came up by itself and rested stiffly across her stomach.

Jane's primary care physician ran imaging tests to rule out structural problems in her hand. None found, he referred her to a movement disorder neurologist.

The neurologist observed slowness and stiffness in her movement (bradykinesia) and impaired fine coordination in her hand. Tentative diagnosis: Parkinson's disease. Jane was put on a dopamine precursor (Sinemet) for a 3-month trial. Her symptoms improved. Parkinson's diagnosis confirmed. Shortly thereafter, her neurologist changed her therapy to a dopamine agonist, which was to be her drug of choice for the next seven years.

Jane's neurologist did not give her any literature or education about the disease. Since she did not know anyone who had Parkinson's, the diagnosis did not upset her. As far as she was concerned, a little handwriting problem and her right-arm action when she walked had little impact on her. Pop a pill and the issue was minimized. No reason to fret over it, or for that matter, even tell others of her diagnosis.

We had known each other for many years. She was part of my extended family, dating back to when she was in college. Jane was an experienced boater, as was I. In 1998, I decided to retire from a career as a scientist and engineer. I called Jane up one day and told her that I and my Siamese cat, Nefertiti, were going to board my 38-foot trawler (powerboat) and travel down the Intracoastal Waterway from the northern Chesapeake Bay to the west coast of Florida, where we would spend the winter. I asked her if she would like to come. She said yes. We have been together ever since.

For the next six years, we had a great life. We settled in Florida and designed, then built, a home in the waterfront community of Punta Gorda Isles. Jane established a relationship with a local neurologist, whom she saw periodically. All was well, until the year 2005.

In early 2005, Jane began to gain weight, lots of it. She was unable to get a good night's sleep. During the day, she would suddenly fall asleep, even when talking with someone, waking 10 or 20 seconds later as if nothing had happened. By September, she could hardly get around, even with a walker. Getting out of a chair required assistance. She also was exhibiting tremors in her hands and feet. Things were not looking good, but all of this was about to change because of a self-motivated effort to learn more about Parkinson's disease.

In early October of 2005, we went to a Parkinson's seminar. Our initial interest was to learn about deep brain stimulation. However, one of the physicians who spoke discussed the various classes of drugs used to treat the disease, and their side effects. He also spoke of the need for drug therapy to change as the disease progresses. As we drove home, I told Jane, "Make an appointment, we need to talk to your neurologist."

Jane's neurologist discontinued her use of a dopamine agonist. Six months later, she had her life back! She lost 60 pounds and returned to her normal weight. Sleeping became normal with no more dozing off suddenly during the day. No need for a walker. No problem getting up from a sitting position. The tremors and stiffness were still there but otherwise, life was good.

Soon after, I made a startling discovery. From studying the literature, I learned that some people on dopamine agonist therapy develop compulsive behavior. A little snooping uncovered Jane's compulsion. She had been buying fabric. Lots of fabric. More than she would ever use in a lifetime! It was stashed all over the place. No longer on a dopamine agonist, the fabric purchases stopped!

We had recovered from the brink of needing to find Jane a nursing home, all because we became proactive, educating ourselves and being insistent that Jane's medical professionals consider changes in her therapy.

The changes in the drug therapy eliminated the side effects that were prevalent in 2005, but they did not stop the progression of the disease. By the end of 2006, freezing of gait was pronounced, as well as increased slowness of movement, and tremor. Jane could no longer get onto and off a small boat. We sold our boat.

We could not stay away from being on the water. Our solution: go on cruise ships, from the large ocean-going liners to the smaller inland river boats. We found it was the perfect vacation for someone with a disability.

In March of 2010, Jane received her first deep brain stimulator (DBS). She calls the operation a "no brainer" as there was no pain associated with the surgery or post-surgery. The result was spectacular. Tremors were essentially gone on the right side of her body. Involuntary movements called dyskinesia, which can be a byproduct of Parkinson's medication, were greatly reduced. We were so pleased with the result of the surgery that a second DBS was placed in early 2011. Now, both sides of the body were benefitting.

By mid-2011, freezing of gait was lowering our quality of life. Jane did not want to go anywhere. She felt like her feet were glued to the floor. She found she could move her dominant foot up and down, but her brain just would not tell the muscles in her leg to take a step forward. Getting from one side of our home to the other became time-consuming. Time for my inventive mind to step in. I had read that freezing of gait can sometimes be broken by use of a triggering device.

What works for one person may not work for another. One morning, I went into my shop and built something I thought might help. I then stood next to Jane while she tried it out, concerned that either it might not work, or she might fall when she tried to use it. Wow, it worked! It worked great. Off she went! I called my device an ambulator. Jane called it her launcher. She carried her launcher everywhere she went. Life was good again!

Jane's launcher was the solution for walking short distances—a hundred feet or less. For the longer walks, another solution was needed. Time for Jane's first scooter. She called her first one her red spitfire.

Over the next several years we became scooter experts, trying different ones and then settling on a model that weighed only 35 pounds, could be quickly folded into a compact package, yet could easily go 10 miles on a single battery charge.

A breakthrough in Jane's treatment came in 2014. While attending a support group, we learned about "medical centers of excellence." There was such a place for Parkinson's disease only a three-hour car drive from our home. Jane made an appointment. Our first visit lasted more than a day! The result was a comprehensive treatment plan, updated every six months, which has changed our lives for the better.

In the next several years, freezing of gait became worse. Soon, the ambulator and a scooter no longer met the need. More research on mobility devices. Result, a lightweight power wheelchair. I devised a way to easily get the wheelchair into and out of the car. (See Chapter 7 for details about all these devices.)

In 2016, our support group, recognizing that we had learned a lot about Parkinson's disease and its treatment, asked us to give a talk about our experiences. We did so. The word got out and soon we were speaking to support groups on the west coast of Florida (our winter home), eastern Tennessee (our summer home), as well as impromptu small gatherings on cruise ships.

During 2017 and 2018, we gained even more experience managing the disease. Jane suffered several falls, one of which put her in the hospital for three days followed by an additional seven days of rehabilitation in a nursing home. Other treatments included voice therapy, physical therapy, occupational therapy, a urologist, multiple sessions with a psychologist, one meeting with a neurological psychiatrist, and evaluation by a neurological ophthalmologist.

In 2019, we moved to The Villages, Florida, a 55 and over community of 135,000 people, to be near the world-renowned Parkinson's "Center of Excellence," the Norman Fixel Center for Neurological Diseases, located in Gainesville, Florida.

As the reader can see, we have gained 25 years of first-hand experience with Parkinson's disease. Every Parkinson's journey is different, as it is a very personal affliction. However, individual journeys will have similarities, so there is much to learn from those with experience. There are excellent books on the disease, although few that specially focus on practical ideas for how to cope with everyday life, both inside and outside of the home. That is where the focus will be in the remainder of our book.

You may find it worthwhile to keep a computer nearby. We will be sharing links and search terms along the way. You may want to check them out before proceeding to the next subject.

We include photos of assist devices we have found useful. This is not an endorsement by us of any supplier's product(s). We purchased what was available at the time that best met our need. We encourage you to use our experience as a starting point. Do your own research. Make purchase decisions that meet your need.

The best thing you can do to ensure quality of life while coexisting with any disease, is to find and benefit from GREAT medical care. The care we needed, and how we arranged it, is a good place for us to continue our story.

CHAPTER 2 - Obtaining Great Medical Care

If you have been recently diagnosed with Parkinson's Disease (PD), you may not yet appreciate that eventually you may need to be treated by quite a few different medical specialists. In this chapter, we will begin by introducing you to various PD symptoms. We will then define the specialties that treat those symptoms. We will give you descriptions of what they do and share some of our experiences.

Early in our PD journey, we located the specialists we needed, arranged appointments, and sometimes found it necessary to hand-carry reports from one medical practice to another. Eventually, we learned about a nearby PD Center of Excellence. That is where Jane gets her care now. To us, our discovery changed care from good, to great!

We will end this chapter with what we hope will be a convincing argument as to why you should want to be treated by a Center of Excellence as early in your disease progression as possible.

Symptoms

To address how to get great medical care, it is worthwhile listing the various symptoms someone with Parkinson's disease (PD) might encounter during his/her lifetime. For one recently diagnosed, the list below may be discouraging, perhaps downright frightening. On a positive note, it is unlikely one will experience all of them. Many symptoms may not develop until many years after initial diagnosis.

Jane has lived with the disease for 25 years. She has experienced 40% of the following. This is not just a list to us. It is our reality!

- Slowness of movement (bradykinesia)
- Rigidity or stiffness
- Change in handwriting
- Change in facial expression
- Tremors
- Shuffling gait
- Freezing of gait
- Problems with balance
- Difficulty swallowing
- Falls
- Stooped posture
- Reduced small motor function (opening jars, buttoning a shirt)
- Constipation
- Restless leg syndrome

- Dystonia (muscle[s] contracting involuntarily)
- Vision changes; difficulty reading small print
- Loss of smell and/or taste
- Inability to multi-task
- Forgetfulness
- Memory loss
- Speech difficulties; speaking too softly
- Episodes of confusion
- Inability to make even simple decisions
- Losing train of thought
- Problems concentrating
- Cognitive decline
- Depth/spatial perception difficulties
- Insomnia
- Low daytime energy
- Acting out dreams during sleep
- Mood changes
- Urinary incontinence
- Bowel control problems
- Anxiety
- Apathy
- Agitation
- Depression
- Delusions
- Hallucinations
- Dizziness/lightheadedness
- Fainting
- Sensitivity to heat and/or cold
- Sexual dysfunction

Most people, when asked what PD symptoms are, may list only the first half dozen or so. Clearly, the disease impacts far more bodily functions than that. Thus, there will be a need for many types of medical professionals as one's life progresses. We know that from personal experience!

The Patient/Caregiver Team

You may be in a long-term relationship, or you may live alone. When it comes to seeing a doctor or other medical practitioner, it makes no difference. You need someone to go with you to all appointments. We do mean all appointments, regardless of how personal they might be. The best arrangement is for the same person to accompany you each time, be it spouse, life partner, family member or close friend. The two of you comprise a team, a patient/caregiver team.

Some symptoms that can make it difficult for a person with Parkinson's disease (PWP) to have an optimal outcome from a solo visit may be his/her inability to multi-task, and difficulty concentrating, losing train of thought, memory loss and cognitive decline. The caregiver fills in the blanks when needed.

Both parties need to prepare for the appointment. Prepare a list of what topics need to be discussed and what the PWP hopes to realize as an outcome of the visit. Share these early during the visit.

The caregiver makes sure the necessary documentation is taken to the visit: list of drugs, symptoms that need attention, lab work results, medical history and so forth. Do not assume that the doctor will have copies of recent lab work. We have found he/she sometimes does not.

A few years ago, during a six-month visit to Jane's neurologist, the doctor asked her how she was doing. She said, "I am doing fine." I chimed in with a different story, saying "She has declined substantially in the last six months. I have been interviewing nursing homes as I fear her days living at home may be coming to an end." Two hours later, we left the appointment with an action plan that, over the next few months, improved her health so much that a nursing home was no longer in her immediate future. Did having a caregiver attend that appointment make a difference? It sure did!

After a visit, document what was discussed and what is the action plan. This is best done by the caregiver, with review by the PCP. Be thorough. Keep these reports in a place where they can be easily found for future reference. It is far too easy to forget specifics of an appointment, even after a few days. You will find your written report is of substantial value in disease management. If you are not sure what you have written is accurate, send a copy to the doctor and ask that your understanding be verified or corrected.

Keeping Your Own Written Medical History

A great doctor wants to hear your story. Everything. Often, he or she can make a diagnosis just from your story, with poking and prodding, lab tests, and so forth used to confirm the preliminary diagnosis. An important part of your story is your medical history.

We keep our medical histories in written form, which we update frequently. Our histories include the following.

- A title on every page: Medical History of "name of patient"
- Drug allergies
- Drugs that should not be administered (Haloperidol, for example)
- Address and phone numbers
- Email address
- Emergency contacts
- Personal information such as date of birth, marital status, sex, race, religion, language, country of birth, smoker or non-smoker, alcohol consumption, recreational drug use
- Living will, healthcare power of attorney, advanced directive
- Insurance information
- Family medical history: father, mother, siblings
- Physicians: name, address, phone number, specialty (both current and previous)
- Surgeries: types and dates
- Disease history with date(s)
- Eyeglass/contact prescriptions
- Details on any medical implants (deep brain stimulator, pacemaker, other)
- Inoculations: types and dates
- Lab tests: types and dates, results
- Prescription drugs: names, dosages, prescribing physicians, why prescribed, where purchased
- Over-the counter drugs: name, dosage, reason

We find that when we go to a new medical practice, we are given pages of forms to fill out, some which require much of the information listed above. We take a copy of our history, which we tell the receptionist to add to the admission paperwork. That saves a lot of time and assures accuracy. It also primes the doctor with "the story."

Having a copy of your detailed medical history will prove invaluable if you need to suddenly go to the hospital.

Medical Professionals You Will Need

General Practitioner

We believe everyone should establish a solid relationship with a primary care physician (PCP). This is especially true if you have PD. Your PCP is likely the first doctor you will go to if you are not feeling well.

Just because you have Parkinson's does not mean you will not have other health issues. We know that all too well. Jane picked up a lung infection while visiting Central America that had nothing to do with her neurological condition.

We believe in prevention. A thorough periodic physical exam may uncover issues before you are aware of them. Sometimes, those issues can be fixed easily if caught early.

This is not just about the health of the PWP. It is imperative that the caregiver remain healthy. Make sure each of you has a personal care physician as the cornerstone of your medical support team so you can be assured of the best health possible.

In 2012, we went for our annual physical exams. We had known our PCP for years and had a great deal of respect for him. Since we were over age 65, this was to be our annual Medicare exam. He began by apologizing for what was to follow. He said 20-minutes was all that he was authorized to spend with each of us and that part of that would be to ask us a bunch of questions. Do you wear your seatbelt? Do you have a gun in the house? On and on! Then a few pokes and prods, listen to the heart and lungs, and the exam was over. A few weeks later, he informed his patients that he was leaving the practice to join the staff at a prominent hospital. Time to find a new PCP.

We were unhappy with a superficial physical exam. We were also unhappy that at most practices we and our friends were familiar with, it had become difficult to get a prompt appointment and the appointment itself often felt rushed. No wonder—a typical PCP may have 2,000 patients or more!

A friend suggested we consider concierge medicine.

Do an Internet search for "concierge medicine." You will find the definition, and much more.

Here is the definition.

Concierge medicine, also known as retainer medicine, is a relationship between a patient and a primary care physician in which the patient pays an annual fee or retainer. This may or may not be in addition to other charges. In exchange for the retainer, doctors agree to provide enhanced care, including principally a commitment to limit patient loads to ensure adequate time and availability for each patient.

We searched for concierge physicians with a practice in the small town where we lived. We found a doctor that was part of a group called "Medical Doctors Versed in Prevention (MDVIP)."

https://www.mdvip.com/

After an interview with the MDVIP doctor, we decided this was what we were looking for. We signed up. Yes, it costs some money beyond what our insurance pays, but to us it is worth every penny. Our annual physical exams are extensive, with in-depth lab work. We are tested for cognitive function, hearing, lung function, muscle-to-fat ratio, and vision. Then, we benefit from at least an hour with our doctor to discuss our test results, present health, how to improve our nutrition, any near-term actions needed, and so forth. Issues have surfaced that had not yet become symptom-evident, and in each case, were fixable. To us, these findings alone justified the additional cost. Since joining, we have never had to wait more than a day for an appointment. In most cases, we have been seen on the same day. We have our doctor's email address and cellphone number. Yes, we have used both!

For some, the additional cost of concierge medicine may be unacceptable. However, given the many symptoms that those with Parkinson's will need to deal with, having readily available and comprehensive PCP support may prove to be a good investment.

Neurologist

If your PCP suspects you might have a disease of the brain and/or nervous system, you will likely be referred to a neurologist.

If you consider your PCP as one cornerstone of your medical support team, your neurologist will be the other. These two professionals will become two of the most important people in your life. Choose wisely!

The following is from Wikipedia:

Neurologists treat a myriad of neurologic conditions, including stroke, seizures, movement disorders such as Parkinson's disease, autoimmune neurologic disorders such as multiple sclerosis, headache disorders like migraine and dementias such as Alzheimer's disease.
In the United States and Canada, neurologists are physicians who have completed a postgraduate training period known as residency specializing in neurology after graduation from medical school. This additional training period typically lasts four years, with the first year devoted to training in internal medicine. On average, neurologists complete a total of 8-9 years of training. This includes four years of medical school, four years of residency and an optional 1-2 years of fellowship.

A general neurologist may treat more than 100 different conditions, one of which is Parkinson's disease. Neurology is a broad and complex field.

Some neurologists, once they have completed their general training, elect to do two more years of study in a specialty, sometimes referred to as a "fellowship." The study of movement disorders is one example. PD is a movement disorder.

Given a choice, select a movement disorder neurologist as the second cornerstone of your medical team.

Regardless of what kind of neurologist you choose, determine if they work with therapists you will need as your disease progresses. Assure the existence of strong lines of communication between your neurologist and those therapists. If not, you may want to consider other alternatives for treatment.

Movement Disorder Neurologist

The following is from the Michael J. Fox Foundation for Parkinson's Research website:

https://www.michaeljfox.org/

Because they have so much experience treating PD, movement disorder specialists are often best equipped to tailor a plan of care for you and your specific needs. Some people may wait to see a movement disorder specialist until later in their disease course. However, seeing this specialist early in your treatment could help you plan for your care in the future, prepare for potential changes in your Parkinson's and adapt to these changes as they happen. Movement disorder specialists also can connect you with clinical studies to help scientists learn more about Parkinson's and how to treat it.

For those who do not reside in an area that is large enough to justify a full-time movement disorder neurologist, you may need to choose a general neurologist for your care. That does not mean you cannot also associate yourself with a specialist. Ask your general neurologist for a recommendation. You may have to travel occasionally to see the specialist, but it will prove worthwhile, especially as your disease progresses. Those two professionals can work together to optimize your care. We did this for several years.

Speech Therapist

As PD progresses, the power of the PWP's voice may decrease, making it difficult for them to converse with others. As a result, they may become socially withdrawn. Fortunately, there are therapies that can help. Those therapies are the realm of the speech therapist.

You may be able to find a speech therapist in your area who has experience with Parkinson's disease. If not, there are remote treatment alternatives available via Zoom.

See chapter 8 for more detail.

Physical Therapist

The two most common causes of PWP death are pneumonia and falls. The person falls, breaking a hip, the back, or the neck, or injuring the brain. Result: hospitalization, nursing home, decline and then death.

Falls must be avoided. Timely physical therapy may reduce the probability of a fall.

A personal story. Ten years ago, Jane experienced a bad fall. While visiting a neighbor, she lost her balance, falling backward with a loud thump as she hit the floor. Severe pain was almost immediate. An ambulance was called. Concern, a broken hip.

At the hospital, X-rays were taken. The good news, nothing was broken. She had ruptured a blood vessel in her derriere, a true pain in the butt! She was sent home to recover, with instructions to follow-up with her PCP.

Jane's PCP recommended physical therapy targeted at lowering the probability of another fall. We found a physical therapist (PT) who specialized in treating people with movement disorders. He said he would train her body to sense instability and immediately react to right itself.

Jane liked going to her physical therapist. It may have been that he called her "My Lady"!

One therapy was noteworthy. Jane walked backward on a treadmill while wearing what looked like a virtual reality headset. She said she got to watch TV. Of course, all of this was happening while she was in a safety harness.

Success. No more falls. Physical therapy works!

Jane continues to benefit from periodic physical therapy. Sessions are sometimes at the therapist's office and sometimes in our home. Both are proving valuable.

Occupational Therapist

Occupational therapists (OT) are health care professionals who help people maintain or resume their ability to function at home, in the workplace, and in social situations after a medical trauma or due to continuing disability. From a PD perspective, they are especially valuable in helping the PWP and caregiver configure the home to optimize safety.

We had an OT come to our home. She went around with blue tape, marking places where we should install handrails. She also made recommendations on carpeting, aids for working in the kitchen, and so forth.

An OT can help in choice of mobility aids: walkers, scooters, wheelchairs and so forth.

Ask your PCP or neurologist to provide you a prescription for an OT. The service may be covered by your medical insurance.

Later in the book, we will provide more detail on the things our OT recommended as well as some things we came up with on our own.

Swallowing Therapy

The PWP may develop difficulty swallowing. These changes can happen at any time but tend to increase as PD progresses. Just as PD affects movement in other parts of the body, it also affects the muscles in the face, mouth and throat that are used for swallowing.

Difficulty swallowing can lead to malnutrition, dehydration, and aspiration (when food or liquid "goes down the wrong pipe"). Aspiration can lead to aspiration pneumonia, one of the two leading causes of PD death.

We have been fortunate that Jane has not developed swallowing problems. That does not mean she had not been tested. She has, several times. A swallowing test is part of her periodic full PD workup. Why? Because it is imperative that a swallowing issue be discovered well before aspiration happens. Survival rates for aspiration pneumonia are reported at less than 35%!

Swallowing therapy is administered by a speech-language pathologist or a specially trained occupational therapist, targeting the strengthening of swallowing muscles to prevent choking and aspiration. There are specific ways to hold your head when swallowing to avoid aspiration, especially when taking a pill. Your therapist can train you on the correct procedure.

Go to the Parkinson's Foundation website, at https://www.parkinson.org/, click on "Understanding Parkinson's," find "non-movement disorders," and click on "speech and swallowing problems." There, you will find much more on the subject. You can also enter "swallowing" in the search box on the main screen to find podcasts as well as additional information on treatment.

Psychologist/Psychiatrist

Depression and anxiety are quite common in people with PD. Your PCP or neurologist can recommend treatment by a psychologist which may be covered by your medical insurance.

Jane was referred to a psychologist to help her with travel anxiety, especially when traveling on an airliner. She found the stress of the entire airport experience, the boarding and disembarking processes, as well as the flight itself caused her movement disorder to escalate to the point where she just could not function. A few times she had to be carried onto and off the airplane by the flight crew. Unfortunately, a dozen 45-minute sessions with a psychologist did not help. The reason: the issue was never discussed!

When we first met with Jane's psychologist, we suggested that both of us attend some, or perhaps all, sessions. Jane's psychologist refused. Turns out that was a mistake. Jane proved unable to elucidate why she needed help, so the travel anxiety issue was never discussed! Based upon our experience, we recommend that a PD client have their caregiver attend some of the sessions, perhaps every session, at least for the first few minutes, to clearly define the reasons for the PWP being there and to state the desired outcome from the therapy.

A psychologist usually has at least a master's degree, and often a PhD, in psychology. A psychiatrist is a medical doctor who has additional training in psychiatry.

Why might a PWP need to see a psychiatrist? In Jane's case, her movement disorder neurologist made the call. His concern was that the numerous prescription and non-prescription drugs she was taking might produce interactions that could affect her cognitively. A psychiatrist has the knowledge to make such determination and to suggest alternatives where needed. One session was all that was needed. The good news, no issues. However, if there is a change in her drug therapy, another visit may be required.

For a PWP who develops symptoms such as hallucinations, memory loss, episodes of confusion, delusions, agitation, and so forth, the PD treatment team may require the addition of a psychiatrist on a continuing basis.

Urologist

PD can affect the gut and the urinary system. When the urinary system malfunctions, you may need the help of a urologist.

Incontinence is common, especially when PD is advanced.

Another problem PD can cause is a decline in personal hygiene because of degradation in fine motor skill of the hand and arm. This can lead to recurring urinary tract infections (UTIs), especially in women. Recurring infection, with liberal prescribing of antibiotics, may result in drug resistant bacterial strains which can be difficult to treat. If one's PCP is no longer able to cure the UTI, a urologist may need to come to the rescue.

We have a lot of experience with urinary incontinence and recurring UTIs. In chapter 14 we will share solutions that have worked well for us.

Neurological Ophthalmologist

Each of your eyes has six muscles that function to move your eye around. PD can affect these muscles, resulting in vision problems that may be beyond what a general ophthalmologist can treat. You may need a specialist, a neuro-ophthalmologist.

Neuro-ophthalmology is a subspecialty that merges the fields of neurology and ophthalmology.

One thing we learned from Jane's first visit with a neuro-ophthalmologist is that a PWP may not do well wearing variable focus eyeglasses. Her doctor recommended a pair of single-vision glasses for far vision with a second single-vision pair for reading. The alternative was trifocals for general wear. The recommendation you receive may be different.

Make sure you let your eye doctor know you have PD. If your eye doctor is not able to correct your vision to your satisfaction, ask to be referred to a neuro-ophthalmologist.

Centers of Excellence

Let us tell you our story about our first visit to a PD Center of Excellence. We went to the University of Florida (UF) Health Center for Movement Disorders and Neurorestoration at the Norman Fixel Center for Neurological Diseases, located in Gainesville, Florida. At the time of our first visit, we did not realize that this was an international destination for people with movement disorders, such as Parkinson's disease. We were fortunate that it was only a three-hour drive from where we lived.

Once we found out about the Center, Jane called and made an appointment. Today, you will need a referral from your PCP or neurologist to set up the first appointment. Jane was given a date and told that our first visit would last at least one day. Ours ran into the morning of the second day.

After each of Jane's visits, I write a summary of what transpired. The following is an excerpt from that first-visit report.

The Center for Movement Disorders and Neurorestoration is an impressive facility. Absolutely first class! Evaluation was 6 ½ hours in duration. Jane was attended by four neurologists, a nurse-practitioner (deep brain stimulator specialist), and four medical specialists (cognitive evaluator, physical therapist, occupational therapist, and speech therapist). In addition, she received an MRI of the brain. The team would like to see Jane in six months for further evaluation. One additional test that will be run at that time will be swallowing.

Our understanding was that at the end of the day, Jane's medical team met to discuss their findings and they worked together to formulate a treatment plan. The plan was shared with us the following morning.

During subsequent visits, we met with other staff members, including a nutritionist, deep brain stimulator (DBS) surgeon, and a neuropsychiatrist.

The facility offers integrated, interdisciplinary care in movement disorders. Neurologists go there to study for two years to obtain their movement disorder specialty. The center also does research directed at finding ways to lessen disease symptoms with the hope of eventually finding a cure.

We return every six months for testing and evaluation, and now that we live nearby, we go there frequently for specific treatments.

Until we moved to be near Gainesville, we worked closely with a local movement disorder neurologist near where we lived. She had trained at Gainesville, so lines of communication between her and the staff at Fixel were excellent.

There are many PD centers of excellence. Do an Internet search. The following is one result of such a search.

Center of Excellence Network | Parkinson's Foundation

https://www.parkinson.org/expert-care/centers-of-excellence

This site lists 47 medical centers around the world, including 33 in the United States, that the Parkinson's Foundation considers to be Centers of Excellence.

For us, our affiliation with a PD Center of Excellence advanced Jane's PD medical care from good, to GREAT!

If possible, get associated with one of these places for your primary PD care, and do it soon after initial diagnosis. Be willing to travel. Look at any additional cost as an investment in your future!

CHAPTER 3 - Learning from Others

When we were young, there was no Internet. Our World Wide Web was a set of books, called an encyclopedia. Some parents would buy a book a month from a door-to-door salesperson. After a few years, the family would have a complete set that quickly became out of date.

Encyclopedias covered a broad range of topics, with limited detail on any single one. When we needed more information, we went to the local library. Often, the local library did not have what we needed. What followed was a request to another library, with wait times from weeks to months.

Wow, how our world has changed! There is so much information available today that at times it feels overwhelming. Want to know a lot about Parkinson's disease? There are many places learn.

During our 25-year journey, we have interacted with many people with PD. Our observation is that those who have the best quality of life are the ones who have a thirst for knowledge. Sometimes it is the PWP, sometimes the caregiver, and occasionally both. That knowledge is gained from in-person learning, foundations, seminars, publications, and books. It should come as no surprise that a lot of it can be obtained through today's World Wide Web.

In this chapter we will show you how we have educated ourselves, with the hope that you will follow us.

Support Groups

If you are recently diagnosed with Parkinson's disease (PD), you may be hesitant to join a support group. You may initially find the experience depressing. There may be people in wheelchairs; those with noticeable tremor; those who clearly have difficulty moving around; some who look mad all the time; and so forth. Go back and read the symptoms list. It will prepare you. Go anyway. Get over the hesitancy. These people have hopes and feelings, just like you do. They just have PD. Get to know them. You will develop close and lasting friendships, while you learn from them.

We have participated in many support groups. The ones we have found most valuable have been those that are open to both men and women and that have two different types of meeting formats, often alternating month-to-month.

The first format is a guest speaker invited to speak to the entire group. That person may be a professional, or perhaps a lay person like us. Topics do not need to always be medical.

The second format is just for the people with Parkinson's (PWP) and caregivers. The meeting begins with everyone present and then quickly splits into two groups: those with PD, and the caregivers. It helps to have a moderator for each group, but most of the interaction comes from the people present. There is a lot to be learned here. Your peers have a lot of knowledge which, with a little effort, you can get them to share.

A word of caution: people seem to love sharing what drugs they are taking. Listen, but do not act. It is easy to purchase the latest over-the-counter miracle cure only to find a serious interaction with what you already take. Drug therapy needs to be personalized by the PWP's medical team. All drugs should be considered, both prescription and non-prescription!

Where can you find the nearest Parkinson's support group? Check community publications. Ask your medical team. Try an online search for support groups in your area. Call a physical therapy and/or occupational therapy clinic and ask them. A nearby hospital may provide a lead. If you have the web application in your area called "Nextdoor" (https://nextdoor.com), establish an account and post a request for information on local support groups.

Suppose there is no support group in your area. Start one. No need to be a PD expert. In fact, no need to even have Parkinson's disease. If you can arrange a meeting location and get out the word, people will come! One support group to which we belonged was led by a caring individual who did not have PD, did not even have a spouse or family member who had PD, but saw a need in his community. It evolved into a wonderful group of people.

We have benefitted significantly from attending support groups. Already mentioned is how we learned of Centers of Excellence. In later chapters of this book, we will introduce other things we learned. One was Parkinson's foundations, which is our next topic.

Parkinson's Foundations

Parkinson's foundations are a rich source of information.

The following are ones we use:

Parkinson's Foundation   https://www.parkinson.org/

Michael J. Fox Foundation   https://www.michaeljfox.org/

Davis Phinney Foundation for Parkinson's   https://davisphinneyfoundation.org/

American Parkinson Disease Association   https://www.apdaparkinson.org/

Neuro Challenge Foundation for Parkinson's   https://www.neurochallenge.org/

Some of these foundations have local groups. Check their websites to see if there is a group near you.

Programs and Seminars

The Parkinson's foundations listed in the previous section offer both in-person and remote educational programs and seminars. Check their websites. You will find a library of previous sessions as well as those scheduled for the future.

Publications

We recommend the first printed materials you add to your Parkinson's library are free pamphlets published by the Parkinson's Foundation. Each pamphlet is about 50 pages long and a quick read. To find them, go to the Parkinson's Foundation website, https://www.parkinson.org/, and follow the path: Living with Parkinson's Disease/Resources and Support/ Order Publications. You can also download PDF versions or get electronic versions for your Kindle book reader.

The following is what is available. If you read only one, read the "Frequently Asked Questions - A Guide to Parkinson's Disease." It will put you on the road to becoming an expert!

- Frequently Asked Questions – A Guide to Parkinson's Disease
- Living Your Best Life - A Guide to Parkinson's Disease
- Fitness Counts – A Guide to Parkinson's Disease
- Speech and Swallowing - A Body Guide to Parkinson's Disease
- Surgical Options – A Treatment Guide to Parkinson's Disease
- Managing PD Mid-Stride – A Treatment Guide to Parkinson's Disease
- Sleep – A Mind Guide to Parkinson's Disease
- Mood – A Mind Guide to Parkinson's Disease
- Cognition – A Mind Guide to Parkinson's Disease
- Psychosis – A Mind Guide to Parkinson's Disease

While you are at the above site, you may want to order a copy of the "Newly Diagnosed Kit."

We subscribe to *Brain and Life* magazine. The subscription is free.

https://www.brainandlife.org/

Consider a donation to organizations that provide publications and magazines at no cost. They rely on donations to fund their work and to supply materials to those who are unable to afford them.

Books

There are many PD books. Go to Amazon.com/books and do a subject search. Usually, you can read the first few pages of a specific book to see if the content interests you.

When Jane began her treatment at the Norman Fixel Center for Neurological Diseases, her lead neurologist was Dr. Michael S. Okun. Dr. Okun has authored or co-authored four PD books. All four are in our library.

- *Parkinson's Treatment - 10 Secrets to a Happier Life*, Michael S. Okun, M.D.
- *10 Breakthrough Therapies for Parkinson's Disease*, Michael S. Okun, M.D.
- *Ask the Doctor about Parkinson's Disease*, Michael S. Okun, M.D., Hubert H. Fernandez, M.D.
- *Living with Parkinson's Disease – A Complete Guide for Patients and Caregivers*, Dr. Michael S. Okun, M.D., Irene A. Malaty, M.D., Wissam Debb, M.D.

Here are a few more books we have in our library.

- *The Muhammad Ali Parkinson Center 100 Question and Answers about Parkinson's Disease*, Abraham Lieberman, M.D.
- *Every Victory Counts*, Davis Phinney Foundation, Monique Giroux, M.D., Sierra Farris, PA-C, IPAS, plus 40 other contributors. Order directly from the Foundation.
- *300 Tips for Making Life Easier, Parkinson's Disease*, Second Edition, Shelly Peterman Schwarz

Educational Courses

For those of you who want to broaden your medical knowledge beyond PD, check out "Great Courses." Courses are available on DVD or by streaming through their service called "Wondrium."

- The Great Courses   https://www.thegreatcourses.com/
- Wondrium   https://www.wondrium.com/

We have taken more than 40 courses through these two services. Many were not specific to medicine, though some were. We have found that by increasing our understanding of how the human body works, we are better able to talk to our doctors. Here are a few titles we have enjoyed.

- Understanding the Human Body: An Introduction to Anatomy and Physiology
- The Human Body: How We Fail, How We Heal
- Medical School for Everyone – Emergency Medicine
- Medical School for Everyone – Grand Rounds Cases
- An Introduction to Infectious Diseases
- The Neuroscience of Everyday Life
- Understanding the Brain
- The Science of Integrated Medicine

- Practicing Mindfulness: An Introduction to Meditation
- Nutrition Made Clear

The Great Courses run sales often with significant savings. Get on their mailing list.

We have a yearly subscription to the Wondrium streaming service which we find to be cost effective.

Another reason for taking courses, reading books, attending seminars and so forth is that you need to keep your brain active. That is certainly true for PD, but it applies to caregivers as well. We live in a wonderful time, where information is readily available. Exercise your brain.

You also need to exercise your body. Physical exercise is proven to slow the progression of PD. That will be our next topic.

CHAPTER 4 - Exercise

General

Exercise is good for all of us. What exercise is best for you? That which you do!

Exercise may reduce the rate of progression of Parkinson's disease. You may see a slower rate of decline—or even improvement—in the following:

- Gait and balance
- Flexibility and posture
- Motor coordination
- Endurance
- Working memory and decision making
- Attention and concentration
- Quality of sleep

While any exercise is good, there are specific programs targeted at PD. What you want to strengthen is the connection between your brain and muscles. Do exercises which involve both thinking about how to move and directing that movement.

Parkinson's Specific

Ballroom dancing is reported to be excellent for those with Parkinson's disease (PD). Both of us are of the "two left feet" persuasion, so we never got into it. For those who do not have significant movement disorder, it is an activity worth pursuing. Not only does it strengthen the brain and muscle connection, but it is a wonderful social activity as well.

As mentioned in Chapter 1, we live in a retirement community of 135,000 people, most over the age of 55. It has been reported that in the USA, 1% of the population over the age of 60 have PD. So, no surprise that our community has several support groups and exercise alternatives. Dance is one of them, typically 45 minutes per session which is choreographed to music. Check your community—perhaps a PD dance program is available in your area. If not, why not start one?

There is a nationwide PD program called "Big and Loud." Big and Loud therapy is designed to improve the motor symptoms in people with Parkinson's disease, specifically, movement and speech. It is called "LSVT Big." The focus is to overcome the problem of movement so that the PWP moves faster and walks with bigger steps. The program may be available in your area.

LSVT Big may be offered in a group setting or one-on-one. Jane has benefitted from the one-on-one therapy at a physical therapy center. Is it exercise? Jane can tell you it is. She would come home from a session, worn-out from moving around.

Search "LSVT Big" to learn more.

https://www.lsvtglobal.com/LSVTBig

Another PD-specific exercise program is called "Rock Steady Boxing." We do not have first-hand experience with the program but know people who feel they have derived significant benefit from throwing punches!

Do an Internet search for "Rock Steady Boxing."

https://rocksteadyboxing.org

The Parkinson's Foundation website says to call 1-800-473-4636 to find exercise classes in your area. Check out the following link.

https://www.parkinson.org/pd-library/fact-sheets/Exercise-and-Parkinsons

Exercise helps, but it is not the only PD therapy you will need. You will be taking pills. We have some experience with PD drugs that is worth sharing.

CHAPTER 5 - Drugs

We are not physicians or medical professionals. We are not qualified to discuss specific drugs or drug therapy. There are plenty of readily available reference materials with which you can educate yourself, some which are listed in chapter 3, Learning from Others.

Your medical team, which includes you, should have the final say on what drugs you take, dosage(s), and when you take them.

Early in your PD adventure, you may take only a few pills a day. Later, the number and frequency may grow substantially. You will likely need to take some drugs at an exact time. How do you manage that? How can you avoid side effects when prescribed lots of drugs by multiple physicians? These are questions you should want answered.

Experience, and the school of hard knocks, are good teachers. We have learned from both.

Schedule

Jane takes a lot of drugs. At present, 17 different ones. She needs to take a PD pill every two hours, plus or minus 10 minutes! Another drug, once every two weeks. The remainder, once a day with some in the morning and some in the evening.

We both use the plastic pill containers that are readily available from a drug store, general retailer, or on-line seller. They come in different colors and different sizes. We use different color containers for morning and evening pills. Periodically, we load the containers with the pills needed for morning and evening dosing for the next four to six weeks. The process of loading the containers helps us see if a specific drug is getting low and needs to be renewed.

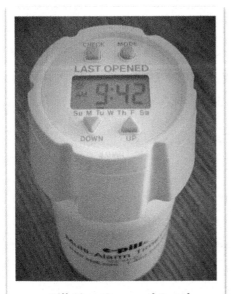

e-Pill TimeCap and Bottle

Assuring that the PD drug be taken on time, every two hours, is more challenging. In Chapter 6, Electronic Gadgets, we will tell you about general-purpose electronic aids we find useful.

There is one device that is electronic and is worth mentioning now. It works great to ensure timely pill consumption. It is a pill bottle cap that knows when the bottle was last opened. It displays the time and day of the week the bottle was last opened. Up to 24 on-the-hour alarms can be set. The display will flash if the bottle was never opened during the set alarm time. We purchased ours through Amazon.com. Search Amazon for "e-Pill TimeCap and Bottle." Local stores may sell it as well.

There are other similar devices, so look around and purchase what works best for you. The device uses a replaceable battery. I put a label on the outside of the bottle with the type of battery required. That way, about a year after purchase, when the battery needed replacing, we did not need to locate the instruction sheet to find out what type of battery to buy.

Side Effects

Most drugs have side effects. Some can be serious.

About 10 years ago, Jane's eye doctor prescribed prescription eye drops for a minor issue. Jane did not tell the doctor that she had PD. When she went to the drugstore, the pharmacist told her he would not fill the prescription. He told her that the eye drops would interfere with one of her PD drugs. The eye doctor, once she was told about Jane's PD, prescribed a different drug.

It is imperative that you let every medical professional you visit know that you have PD. They will be the first line of defense to reduce the chance of medicine side effects.

The second line of defense is to ask your primary care physician (PCP) if a newly prescribed drug will interfere with what you already take. Clear both prescription and over-the-counter drugs. If your PCP is not sure, get the medicine cleared by your neurologist.

The third line of defense is your druggist. However, if you shop around for the best price, and purchase from multiple places, your drug profile may not be in the system and this line of defense may not work.

There is a fourth especially important line of defense—you. Do you read the information that comes with your drugs? You should. Read about the side effects. If there are ones that concern you, talk to your doctor(s). Share the information with each other. There may be side effects that do not become evident to you but might become obvious to another.

Dopamine agonists are known to create obsessive behavior in some people. Some behaviors can destroy a relationship. Others have been reported to destroy a family's financial health. If you are prescribed a dopamine agonist, make sure the caregiver knows of such side effects and that they watch the PWP carefully to detect any that might surface. We know from experience that the PWP may not know they have a problem. The caregiver plays a critical role with this side effect.

Other side effects that we have encountered are disruptions in sleep, excessive and unexplained weight gain, and decreased mobility. Look for these. Talk to your physicians if you experience these. They can reduce your quality of life long before PD does!

Botox

We want to mention one specific drug that has improved Jane's ability to move around, and that is Botox. When you mention Botox to someone, they might think of cosmetic treatment; however, Botox is used to treat many things, one being dystonia.

Dystonia is a movement disorder in which your muscles contract involuntarily, causing repetitive or twisting movements. Jane has significant dystonia in her feet. Her toes involuntary curl up or curl down, for no apparent reason, making it exceedingly difficult for her to walk. It is also painful.

Jane gets periodic Botox injections in the muscles in her feet. The injections are done by her neurologist. The injections relax the muscles, and the toe curl goes away. An injection is good for a few months and then the procedure is repeated.

Ask your neurologist if he or she has experience with Botox injections in the feet. Not everyone does. We know from experience. If the drug is not injected in just the right place, the improvement is minimal or the wearing-off time is reduced.

While traveling, we once went to see a neurologist at a hospital who said he would do her periodic injection. Turns out he had never done it before. Soon, he and another doctor came into the room, carrying a medical book. We think it was *Gray's Anatomy*. They were trying to figure out where to do the injections. This would be the first time they had ever injected Botox into the feet. The injections ended up being painful and short lasting. We never went back!

If your neurologist is not experienced with Botox injections where you need them, ask for a referral. We have had to drive 90 miles on a few occasions to find an experienced person. Now that Jane is treated at a PD Center of Excellence, she gets her shots there. For the Center, this is a routine procedure.

CHAPTER 6 - Electronic Gadgets

Today, there are many electronic devices available that can make life easier. They give access to information and programs that can help you manage Parkinson's disease (PD). In this chapter we will tell you what gadgets we have, how we have enhanced them to make them easier for Jane to use, and what the benefits have been.

Most of the devices we will discuss need access to the World Wide Web, ideally through broadband Internet service in your home. A home system will include a modem and router. Most routers have wireless capability, called Wi-Fi. This allows computers, and other electronic devices, to communicate with one another without the need to run wires all over the house!

Computer

A computer is your window to today's world of information. That should be clear by now. Previous chapters provided Internet links and search parameters for finding valuable information about PD. Many more will follow!

A computer is a valuable tool for staying connected with others. You probably already have an email account. We get a lot of Parkinson's announcements via email since we are on mailing lists for several of the foundations, support groups, and so forth. If you are trying to manage PD and do not have an email account which you check frequently, you are at a disadvantage.

We use an application called Google Calendar to keep track of our appointments. Our two calendars are linked. If Jane makes an entry, it shows on my calendar. The reverse happens as well. That way, we always know what is on our combined schedule.

For those who may not own their own computers, libraries often have some for public use. We recommend you have your own.

While you may choose to take your computer somewhere where there is public Internet access, be aware that security of your personal information may be at risk at such places without stringent electronic safeguards installed and working on your machine.

The most common type of computer in use today is a laptop. Laptops can go where you go, either around the home, or where you travel. Most people have a printer connected to their laptop, either via a cable or Wi-Fi.

A laptop has a small screen, a small keyboard, and a small pointing device, which may not be ideal for someone with PD. Fortunately, there is a fix: connect external devices to your laptop.

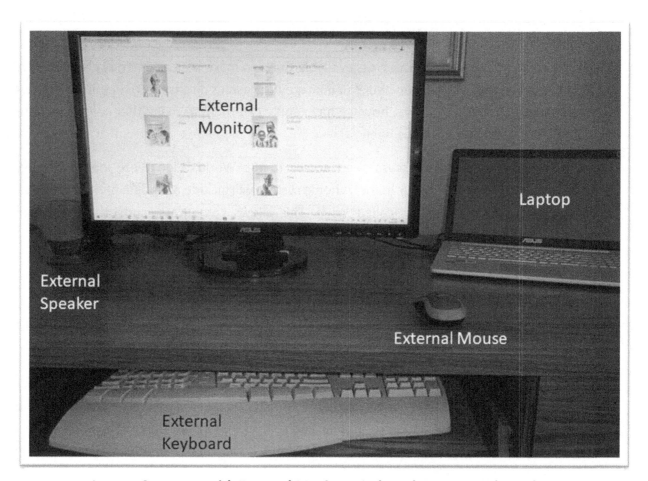

Laptop Computer with External Monitor, Keyboard, Mouse, and Speakers

The photo shows one of our laptop setups. We have connected an external monitor, external keyboard, external pointing device (mouse), and an external sound system (speaker).

Almost any size external monitor can be connected to a laptop computer. Ours are 27 inches, which is far easier for Jane to see detail on than with a 15-inch laptop screen.

External keyboards are readily available. They can be purchased with large print on each key.

One can purchase a trackball or an external mouse as a pointing device. There are many to choose from. Some connect to the laptop with a wire. Others are wireless. We prefer the wireless ones.

It is worth adding an external sound system. Ours have three speakers: left, right, and a woofer. The combination gives us a sound like what you hear from an expensive HiFi system.

One device not shown in the photo is an external camera. We use one for on-line meetings since our laptops, and thus their internal cameras, are tucked away on the corner of our desks. We put the external camera near the external monitor, as needed.

Make sure that your computer has antivirus software installed and operational. Make sure you have selected automatic updates of the operating system so that patches are installed as soon as they become available. These patches often have security updates that protect you from the bad people who roam the World Wide Web.

Back up your files often. Computers do fail. Sometimes, they do so in a way that your precious photographs and documents are gone forever! We use Carbonite, a paid service that continuously backs up our personal files to storage devices located far from where we live. The industry calls this "backing up to the cloud."

Jane once had a catastrophic failure of her computer. Everything on her hard drive was lost. She had not done a local backup for several months. No problem, the computer was replaced, connected to "the cloud," and her information downloaded to her new machine. Nothing lost!

Seek help getting your computer set up if you do not have the skills to do so. Today, there is no shortage of people who can help. Senior centers, the big-box electronics stores, a local computer club, or a neighborhood computer store all are potential sources of help. Of course, you could always enlist the aid of your children or grandchildren!

Smartphone

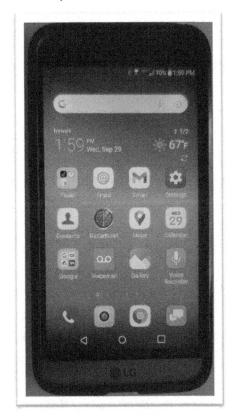

Smartphone

Today, most people have cell phones. Some have abandoned their landline phones and use only their cell phones. A basic cell phone can be used for making and receiving telephone calls and text messages. Some have built-in cameras.

A step up is the smartphone. It is a powerful computer in a small package, but with a small screen. Smartphones have built-in cameras, with performance that rivals expensive dedicated cameras of a few years ago. They also can access thousands of applications, called "apps." Many apps are free, although those normally have imbedded advertisements. Some of the apps are especially useful to someone with PD.

You obtain apps by going to the smartphone's store. For an Android phone, it is called the "Play Store." Apple calls it the "App Store."

If you have a smartphone, try entering "pill reminder" into the app store search engine. You will find several apps that you may want to download and try. It is another alternative for assuring you take your pills on time.

Another app we use frequently is weather radar. You might wonder why this app might be useful for someone with PD. Many of the places we go, including doctor's offices, medical labs, restaurants and so forth, do not have covered entrances to drive under when Jane needs to get out of the car when it is raining. Given that it takes time to get her wheelchair out of the car, and sometimes many minutes for her to get from the car to the chair, she can easily get soaked if it is raining. We use the weather radar app to see what the weather is before we set out. Sometimes, that means leaving early so we arrive in time to get inside before the skies open up!

There are many more apps that are useful to someone with PD. They will be mentioned in future chapters.

Smartphones have excellent cameras. They also can record voice messages. No need for paper and pencil anymore. Want to make a note to yourself? Either speak the note into your phone for later playback or, if it is something that can be photographed, take a picture of it.

Smartphones have Wi-Fi built into them. When at home, no need to use your data allowance to run apps and to access the Internet. You can connect to the Web via your home network.

Smartphones have excellent voice recognition capability. Ask the phone a question instead of trying to type it. Your smartphone is truly a window to the world. We ask our phones questions frequently and we always get a useful response. Try it now. Ask your phone "What is Parkinson's disease"?

Smart Speakers

Examples of smart speakers include Amazon Echo, Google Home Mini, and Apple HomePod. We have several Amazon Echo Dots in our home. We will tell you about ours, which we call Alexa, as an example of how they can provide value to someone with PD.

The following is from Amazon's advertisement:

Amazon Echo, often shortened to Echo, is an American brand of smart speakers developed by Amazon. Echo devices connect to the voice-controlled intelligent personal assistant service Alexa, which will respond when a user says "Alexa." Users may change this wake word to "Amazon," "Echo," "Ziggy," or "Computer." The features of the device include voice interaction, music playback, making to-do lists, setting alarms, streaming podcasts, and playing audiobooks, in addition to providing weather, traffic and other real-time information. It can also control several smart devices, acting as a home automation hub. The smart speaker needs to use Wi-Fi to connect to the Internet as there is no Ethernet port.

Jane has an Echo Dot in her bedroom. She also has an Amazon Smart Plug that her bedside lamp is plugged into. From anywhere in the house, she can say "Alexa, turn on Jane's bedroom light," and the light comes on. When she is in bed and ready to go to sleep, she says "Alexa, turn off Jane's bedroom light." Given that mobility is a problem for Jane, and that she gets around the house in a power wheelchair, this is a real convenience for her as well as an increase in safety.

Smart speakers can be set up as remote monitors, much like a voice-only baby monitor. If the PWP and his/her caregiver sleep in different bedrooms, this is a way to listen in for a call for help.

Cameras

We have installed several Wi-Fi cameras in our home. The cameras work in concert with our smartphones.

One camera is outside, looking down at the front door. When there is a knock at the door, Jane can quickly bring up the front door camera on her smartphone, to see who is there. She can also speak to the person at the door via the camera's voice microphone and speaker system. That way, she can let them know that it may take her a few minutes to get to the door. Otherwise, they might leave, believing no one is home. She also finds it useful to see if a package has been left by the front door.

CHAPTER 7 - How to Unfreeze

In chapter 1, we explained that Jane's freezing of gait became a significant issue by mid-2011. It had lowered our quality of life as she did not want to go anywhere. She felt like her feet were glued to the floor. She found she could move her dominant foot up and down, but her brain just would not tell the muscles in her leg to take a step forward. I came up with a solution which I

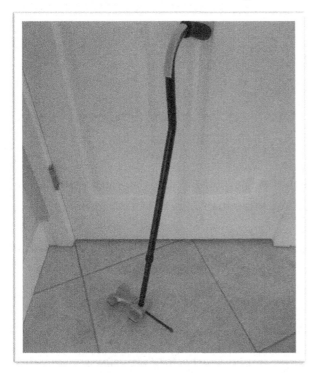

Ambulator/Launcher

called an "ambulator." Jane called it a "launcher." It consisted of a purchased cane into which I drilled a hole to insert a short length of aluminum rod. At the end of the rod, I attached a plastic tip which I bought at a hardware store. Total cost, less than $30.

Jane used the cane as a triggering device to get herself moving. She would put the short horizontal piece in front of her foot and her eye/brain would see it as an obstacle that she needed to step over. Off she would go. Once underway, she rotated the cane a quarter turn so that she would not trip over the horizontal piece as she continued to walk. When she would freeze again, she would repeat the process. This simple device significantly improved our quality of life.

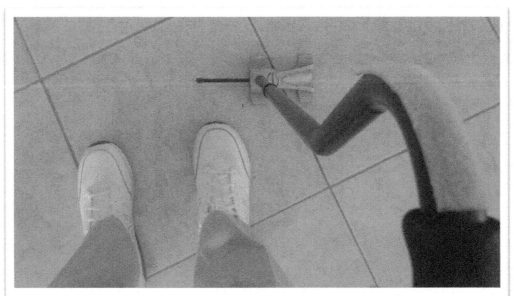

The Need to Step Over an Obstacle Acts as a Walking Trigger

Today, we look back and are utterly amazed that until Jane began getting treatment at a Parkinson's Center of Excellence, the idea of a triggering device was never mentioned to us. In fact, one of Jane's neurologists, who was not a movement disorder specialist, saw the ambulator and asked the purpose. I provided a little education!

Today, there is good news. There are plenty of references on triggering devices. Not every device works for everyone. Our experience is that you need to try different ones and see what works best for you.

Here are a few of the triggers that we are aware of:

- Laser pointer – point it at the floor in front of you, and step on it.
- Use a metronome. Go to your smartphone store. Enter "metronome" to find a free app. Adjust the speed as needed. Use an earbud so others do not have to listen to tick, tick, tick!
- Listen to marching music. Check your smartphone store for an app. The music app called Pandora has many music choices, including marching music.
- Try counting 1, 2, 3, go.
- We have been told that some people with Parkinson's step backward, and then step forward.

Especially important: do not try these alternatives by yourself. There is a risk of falling. Work with someone. A physical therapist would be the perfect choice.

For more information on triggering alternatives, do an online search for "Freezing of Gait and Parkinson's Disease" or "Freezing and Parkinson's." You might also try the following URLs:

https://www.apdaparkinson.org/article/freezing-gait-and-parkinsons-disease/

https://parkinson.org/sites/default/files/Freezing-and-Parkinsons.pdf

CHAPTER 8 - Speaking Loudly and Clearly

Over time, a person with Parkinson's (PWP) often loses his/her ability to talk in a normal voice, making it hard for others to hear him/her. He/she does not even know he/she is speaking softly. A battle ensues between the PWP and his/her caregiver. The PWP tells the caregiver he/she has become hard of hearing. The caregiver tells the PWP to speak up. We went through this.

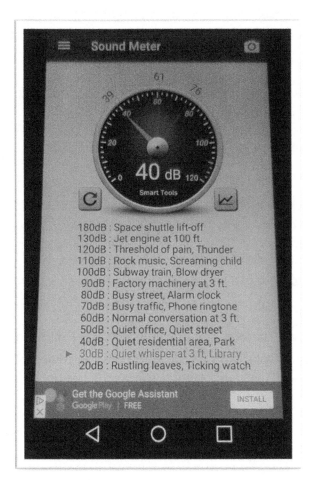

Smartphone Sound Meter

I devised a method to find out who had the problem, so we would know who needed to seek a professional.

My solution was to get a device that measures the volume of sound, such as speech, and then measure each of us talking at what we thought was normal conversational voice level. Fortunately, it proved quite easy to make the measurements. Smartphone to the rescue!

We found a free app for our Android phone called "Sound Meter." It is likely available for an Apple phone as well. Do a search as there are a number of these type apps available. Choose what looks like it will work best for you.

We set the smartphone equidistant between the two of us and we took turns talking. After one of us talked, we recorded the sound meter reading. Then, we reset the meter and the other person talked. The absolute reading was not important, only the differences in readings for each of us. Conclusion, my hearing was fine.

Jane was talking so softly that the sound meter did not go up far. She was the problem!

In Chapter 4, we introduced the Big and Loud program. it may be offered in your area either one-on-one or in a group setting. In addition to emphasizing movement, it also concentrates on speaking loudly. The links to the program are in Chapter 4.

We did not have the Big and Loud program available where we lived. Fortunately, we had a great alternative called Voice Aerobics®.

Voice Aerobics® is a whole-body voice strengthening program developed to focus on posture, breathing and voice. Mary Spremulli, the brains behind the program, is a medical speech-language pathologist located in Punta Gorda, Florida.

Mary worked one-on-one with Jane. After the course of treatment, Jane spoke in a normal voice, and she speaks so even to this day!

While we were working with Mary, she was in the process of developing a gadget that the PWP would wear on his/her wrist which would flash a subtle LED light when he/she was speaking at a normal level. That device, HI-VOLT® voice-on-light, is now fully commercialized.

Mary Spremulli provides speech therapy via telepractice, as well as on-site. She also has products, such as DVDs, which can be purchased for home use.

Search the Internet for "Voice Aerobics" or enter the following link into your computer's browser: https://voiceaerobicsdvd.com/

There may be other speech-language pathologists who offer therapy via telepractice or in your area. Ask your neurologist for a recommendation/referral.

If you get your Parkinson's treatment at a Center of Excellence, they likely have a Parkinson's voice specialist on staff to provide the treatment you need. If you do not have a voice specialist where you live, treatment via telepractice may be an alternative worth pursuing.

We believe it is important that this issue be dealt with as soon as it becomes evident. Failure to address the problem may result in the PWP withdrawing from social situations, and lines of communication between him/her and the caregiver may be seriously damaged.

CHAPTER 9 - Making the Home Parkinson's Friendly

The home can be a dangerous place for a person with Parkinson's disease (PWP). Falling is common. Jane has fallen multiple times. Two falls put her in the hospital. Fortunately, she was not seriously injured. The falls were a wake-up call. We needed to make our home as Parkinson's friendly as possible.

In this chapter we will share with you some of what we did to make our home PD friendly. In Chapter 10, The Bathroom, and in Chapter 11, The Bedroom, we will go into greater detail. To a person with PD, the bathroom and the bedroom are so important for personal safety that these rooms deserve a chapter all their own!

After Jane's second fall, her doctor gave her a prescription for an occupational therapist (OT) to visit our home. The OT made multiple recommendations. She walked around the house with a roll of blue masking tape in her hand, marking where grab bars needed to be installed. Grab bars and handrails are at the core of making a home PD friendly.

Grab Bars

In chapter 10 we will discuss grab bars in the bathroom, an obvious place to put one. That is not the only place for them. Put them wherever the PWP might need something sturdy to hold onto when moving about.

Installing a grab bar, or a handrail, is something the home craftsman might do, providing the job is done correctly. The devices must be screwed into wall studs or, in some cases, concrete block. Attaching it to drywall is unacceptable. A grab bar that pulls out when used is worse than no grab bar at all.

Some homes have metal wall studs instead of wooden ones. Metal studs require special fasteners to ensure that grab bars are rigidly attached.

The photo shows the entry way from the garage into the living quarters at the home we owned a few years ago. This home did not prove to be PD friendly. Living quarters were on multiple levels. To get from the garage to the living quarters required going up a flight of stairs. I added grab bars in several places. The photograph shows what I did so that Jane

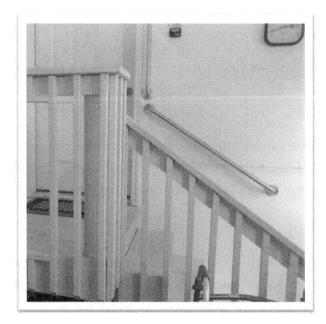

Grab Bars and Hand Railings

could safely get from the living quarters to the garage and back. Although Jane had trouble walking due to freezing of gait, she was able to go up and down steps, provided she had something secure to hold.

During our 25-year PD experience, we have lived in three different homes. We sold the above home as it did not meet our needs as Jane's PD progressed. We had multiple grab bars installed in the other two homes. Both homes were in Florida retirement communities, where there are lots of seniors. In both places we were able to locate contractors who did nothing but install grab bars and handrails. We had them install what we needed since we had to deal with both metal studs and drilling through tile. I felt it was time for a professional!

Area Rugs

We have owned homes with carpeted rooms, hardwood floors and tile floors. An injury from a fall in a room with carpeting might be less severe than a fall onto a solid surface. The downside is that carpeting, especially thick carpeting, may increase the chance of a fall for someone with PD. Look to an OT for advice about what type of flooring is best for you, since every case of PD is unique.

Our current home is tile throughout. Our OT feels this is ideal, given that Jane now spends much of her day in a power wheelchair. To us, lack of area rugs makes the place feel cold, almost institutional. We are unwilling to give up our area rugs. The solution: double-sided carpet tape.

Double sided carpet tape is readily available on-line or locally. The tape comes in two-inch width, 30 yards long. The tape is attached to the floor by removing the protective layer from one side and then pressing it into place. Next, remove the top protective layer and press the area rug into place.

The carpet tape has worked well for us. Jane's power wheelchair moves smoothly over the area rugs. She can use her walker to navigate the rugs as they do not slip or get caught up in the walker legs.

One concern we had was ease of tape removal. In heavily traveled areas, we find the adhesive eventually degrades and the tape needs to be replaced about every six months. To our pleasant surprise, we found that the old tape easily peels away from both the floor and the carpet.

Door Guards

If you eventually need to get around the house with a wheelchair, or you find it necessary to use your foot to kick open a door, the door will suffer. Best to install door guards before damage happens. We know this from experience!

Metal door guards, called push plates, are available at hardware stores or on-line. Do an Internet search for "stainless steel push plates." They come in various sizes. Install them by drilling several holes in the door, and then screw the plate to the door.

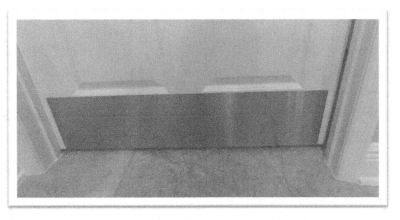

Metal Door Guard

The photo shows one of the push plates in our current home. If the plate were removed, you would see a big hole which Jane punched into the door while she was learning to drive her power wheelchair!

Be forewarned, better to install the push plates before you need them.

When you want to sell your home, the plate adds a nice touch to the door, or if the buyer does not want the plate, remove it, patch the small screw holes with putty and add a coat of paint. No need to replace the entire door, providing you installed the plate before it was needed!

Extending Your Reach

Jane has found three devices useful for reaching things when her limited mobility makes it difficult to do so without assist.

One useful device is called a "grabber reacher tool." They come in different lengths. Squeeze the handle of the tool to activate a pair of grippers located at the other end of the tool.

Jane finds a "back scratcher" useful to have around the house. She uses it to pull things towards her, adjust the window blinds, adjust placemats on the dining room table, and so forth. They can be purchased fixed length or adjustable.

She says a stick with magnet on the end is a useful tool for retrieving small things that are made of ferrous metal. The sticks can be purchased fixed length or telescoping.

Nightlights

Light Emitting Diode (LED) nightlights have come way down in price in the last few years. They last for a long time; put out plenty of light; come on automatically at night; and require a miniscule amount of electricity. Do an Internet search for "LED night lights" to find where to purchase. Buy more than one! Put them all over the house. At night, a small amount of light in hallways, bathrooms, the kitchen, and so forth, will reduce the chance of someone falling when he/she gets up in the middle of the night to raid the refrigerator or to visit the bathroom.

Wheelchair Ramp

Jane went many years before she needed a scooter, then a wheelchair. During her scooter days she was able to walk into and out of our home with the help of a walker. Once a wheelchair became necessary, we needed solutions for navigating across door thresholds. Some of the door thresholds we encounter are only 5/8 inches high which are easily crossed in either a manual or electric chair. The threshold out to our patio is 3 ½ inches high. For that, we needed to add a ramp.

We purchased an aluminum ramp from an on-line store. Do an Internet search for "wheelchair ramp for homes." You will find plenty of sources, both on-line and at the big-box retail outlets.

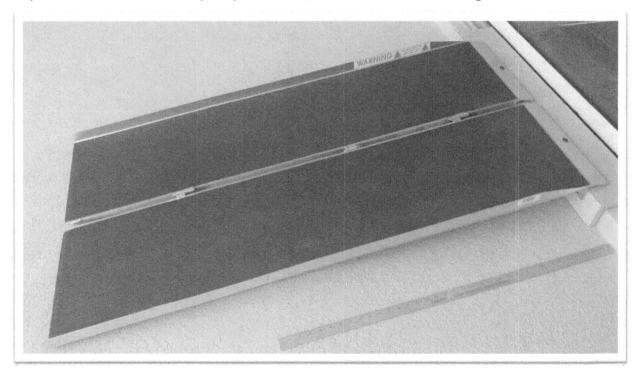

Aluminum Wheelchair Ramp

The ramp shown in the above photo has a 3 ½ inch rise in a 5-foot run. Jane drives her electric wheelchair up and down the ramp with no risk of falling.

If you decide to build your own ramp, you need to understand what incline is safe. It is called rise over run—how many inches of rise, maximum, is appropriate for each foot of ramp length. A good reference is the America with Disabilities Act (ADA) ramp standards. It states that ramp slope must be no steeper than 1:12 (1 inch of vertical rise to 12 inches of ramp length).

Search the Internet for "ADA Ramp - ADA Compliance" for more detail.

https://www.ada-compliance.com/ada-compliance/ada-ramp

Suppose the door from your garage to your home's living quarters is four feet above the garage floor. Per the ADA guidelines, the ramp would have to be 48 feet long! That is what we faced with our previous home. A ramp was not going to work. Next alternative was an expensive power lift. Given other challenges of Jane living in a multi-level home, we decided to move!

Buying a Home

Once someone is diagnosed with PD, it is time to consider if one's existing home is PD-friendly, or if it can be modified to be so. The home as is, may be fine for many years. However, in time, as PD symptoms become more significant, home renovation may be needed. Renovation should be anticipated and accomplished in advance of need. Do not wait until a fall tells you it is time to act.

Your current home may not be easily changed to meet the need of someone that lives in a wheelchair. A multi-level home may be especially challenging.

In early 2019, we decided it was time to sell our multi-level home and buy something that would be Parkinson's friendly. Our criteria for the home included the following:

- Ground level, single floor
- Low exterior door thresholds
- Solid surface floors throughout
- Garage large enough for a minivan with side wheelchair access
- Roll in shower
- Thirty-six inch width exterior doors with lever knobs
- Interior pocket doors wherever possible
- Hallways wide enough for easy navigation by electric wheelchair

We focused on retirement communities in Florida which were no more than an hour's drive from a Center of Excellence for PD. A community of active, age 55 and older folks, which offered opportunity for recreational and social interaction was important to us. Our choice, The Villages, a retirement community of 135,000 people, is located just west of Leesburg, Florida. The Villages, by car, is one hour south of Gainesville, where the Fixel Institute for Movement Disorders is located.

We looked at many homes, of various sizes and floor plans. Some homes were not acceptable for us as the hallways were too narrow or it was nearly impossible for Jane to maneuver her electric wheelchair from the living area into the bedroom. Some floor plans were well designed to assure privacy between sleeping quarters and the main living area, but with the result that the homes were not disability friendly. After a week of looking, with no solution found, we returned home to wait for our real estate agent to call us and tell us he had found the perfect home. He did!

We purchased an existing home that, when it was built, had been customized for a gentleman who was a quadriplegic. The home had the features we sought.

The front door and the door into the garage have low thresholds. To keep rain from coming in under the front door, the front walkway had been graded as a wheelchair ramp with the surface made of paver brick. Very clever!

Most of the interior doors are pocket with a passage width between thirty inches and thirty-five inches. Hallways are mostly forty-eight inches wide with only a few at thirty-six inches.

The home already had grab bars in strategic areas, but we added more. We replaced some of the towel racks with grab bars so that they could serve a dual purpose.

Is our home perfect for someone with advanced PD? No, but it comes close.

If you are considering building a home, you will be able to fine-tune the design to make it PD perfect.

Do an Internet search for "Disability Home Design." You will find several links that are rich with design information. The following one is worth examining:

https://disabilitysmartsolutions.com/AccessibilityConsulting/disability-home-design/

This site has a long list of things one should consider when designing a handicap friendly home. For example, in addition to what we have in the home we purchased, it is recommended that doors throughout a handicap home be three feet wide, hallways be five feet wide, and there be a covered outdoor entryway. These are just a few of the recommendations.

For a new home, or a home renovation, it is imperative that the bathroom be configured to accommodate the PWP. That is the subject of the next chapter.

CHAPTER 10 - The Bathroom

The most dangerous room in the home is the bathroom. A few statistics from the Center for Disease Control (CDC).

- Every year around 234,000 people slip in the bathroom
- 79% of bathroom injuries occur to people ages 65 and older
- 33% of elderly who fall in the bathroom need hospitalization
- One person dies every day by using a bathroom or shower

Add Parkinson's disease (PD), and the likelihood of a bathroom fall is greater.

In this chapter we will describe what steps we have taken to make the bathroom a safe place for Jane.

The Shower

The photo below is of one of our bathroom showers. There are two grab bars. The size and location were defined by an occupational therapist (OT). They were professionally installed to assure they were securely attached to the wall studs.

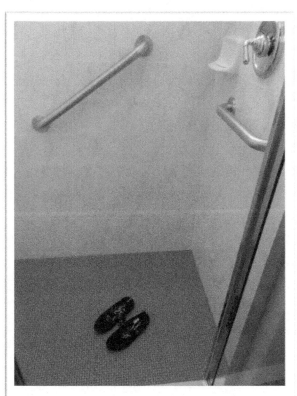

The shower floor has interlocking rubber tiles that we purchased from Amazon.com. They are 11½ inches on each side and can be snapped together. Individual tiles can be easily cut with a utility knife or shears. It only took a few

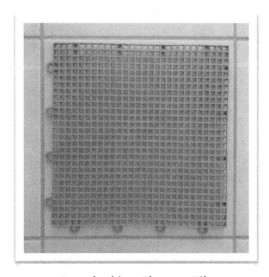

Shower with Grab Bars, Rubber Floor Mat and Shower Shoes

Interlocking Shower Tile

minutes to configure tiles to totally cover the shower floor. Do an Internet search for "interlocking rubber floor tiles."

Jane wears pool shoes whenever she sets foot into the shower.

Not shown is a seat. This shower has a built-in seat. Shower chairs are readily available if your shower does not have a built-in seat.

We added a shower head with a handheld attachment. The handheld wand has a receptacle that slides up and down on a rail which allows it to be adjusted to a height that works best for Jane. She can remove the wand and use it to shower specific parts of her body.

The shower head combination shown has a valve that can be adjusted for shower head only, wand only, or both on simultaneously.

A shower should be large enough to accommodate two people. A person with Parkinson's disease may need help in the shower room. Decreased mobility, the need to be seated, and the requirement to always hold onto a grab bar may make it difficult for to get fully bathed alone. For a couple, it can be a fun time as well!

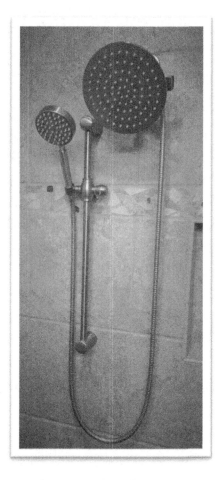

Shower Head with Handheld Attachment

The Toilet

A raised toilet seat with handles may prove a good investment. It can make it much easier for a PWP to get up after completing his/her task. Some people with PD find that a foot stool that raises the feet while on the toilet helps the body function properly. For tens of thousands of years, humans defecated by squatting. A toilet seat is a modern invention and not ideal for someone with an unruly digestive system. PWPs often have unruly digestive systems.

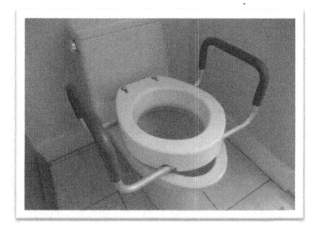

Raised Toilet Seat

Bidet

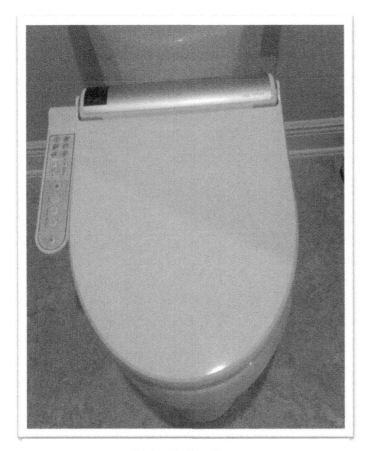

Bidet Toilet Seat

Jane went through a period of recurring urinary tract infections (UTIs).

Urinary tract infections can be serious if they are untreated as they may spread to the kidneys, resulting in a life-threatening condition.

Recurring UTIs may encourage drug resistant bacteria. A normal course of antibiotics by mouth may not cure the infection. An IV may be necessary and even then, getting rid of the bacteria may be challenging.

Personal hygiene when using the toilet can be challenging for those with PD. It sets the stage for UTIs, especially for women.

When Jane was dealing with recurring UTIs, her doctor told me to put in a bidet toilet seat. I did. Jane loves it. I love it. Jane's UTI issue quickly got under control!

Years ago, a bidet was a separate device from the toilet. Today, a toilet seat can be removed and replaced by a bidet toilet seat. Connect the seat to electricity and water and you will immediately learn why Asians and Europeans have been using bidets for so long!

Do an Internet search for "bidet toilet seat." You will find many choices and various price-points.

Our recommendation is not to skimp when you buy your seat. Get one that heats the water. A heated seat is a treat on cold mornings! Stainless steel fittings are better choice than plastic. We spent about $600 for our seat when we purchased it in 2018. Worth every penny!

Seats can be purchased with the controls built into the seat as shown in the photograph. You can also buy one with a remote control. The remote might be useful if the caregiver needs to participate in the PWP's toileting activity.

CHAPTER 11 - The Bedroom

In the early years of our Parkinson's experience, there was no need to do anything special to the bedroom. As Jane's mobility became more challenging, that changed. Today, she has difficulty getting into and out of bed. We came up with three easy-to-implement solutions. She also finds it challenging to get to the bathroom in time. There was an easy fix for that as well.

Bed Height

The average height of a bed in North America is 26 inches. We have observed that there has been a trend toward thicker mattresses and box springs. Heights of as much as 36 inches or more are not that uncommon. We purchased a bed for our guest room; its height is 36 inches! Way too high for someone with PD.

We searched the Internet and found that a mattress should come to one's knee joint. However, for someone with a disability, 21 inches is recommended.

Jane's current mattress is 26 inches high. She uses a step to make it easier for her to get into and out of bed. A 21-inch mattress height may be in our future!

Do an Internet search for "bed steps for adults." You will find many choices, some with handrails. We have several, with handrails and without. Jane uses what works best for her at the time.

When you go shopping for a new bed (or just a mattress and box springs), take a tape measure with you so you can assure yourself that you are not about to purchase something that is too high. Ask the bedding store if they can supply a frame that allows the bedding you choose to be at the desired height.

While a fancy bed with side boards, a headboard, and a footboard may look nice, it may not be the best choice for someone with PD. A simple frame with a headboard may be a better choice.

Bed Rails

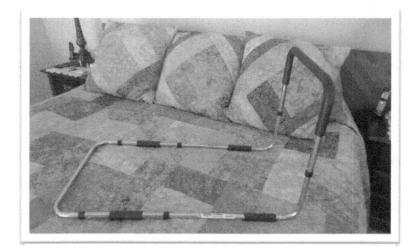

Bed Rail Assembled and Ready to Install

Those with Parkinson's disease may develop sleep disorders where they flail around or act out their dreams. A fall out of bed is not uncommon. Side rails are readily available that reduce the chance of rolling out of bed. They will also help the PWP to get into and out of bed.

The first photo shows what we use, assembled and ready to install. The device slides between the mattress and box springs.

The second photo shows the rail installed on one side of the bed.

Purchase two rails, one for each side.

Do an Internet search for "adult bed rail." You will find many choices. There are rails that fold up so that they can be taken along when traveling.

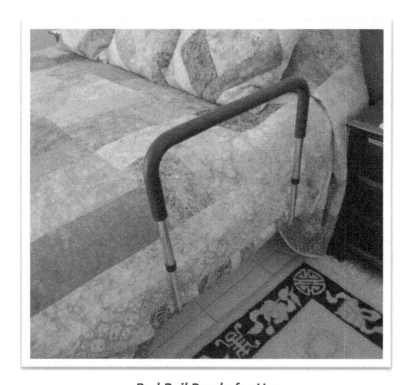

Bed Rail Ready for Use

Jane has a bed rail bag attached to one of her rails. Into the bag she puts drugs she may need at night, the TV remote, smartphone, back scratcher for reaching things, and so forth. She purchased hers on Amazon.com. Do a search for "bed rail bag."

Ladders

We are old enough to remember when people who lived in two-story homes kept a rope ladder in second floor bedrooms. In the event of a fire, the rope ladder was tied to something sturdy and then dropped out the window. The ladder was used to safely get out of the house when no other means of egress was available. You may remember these from your early life!

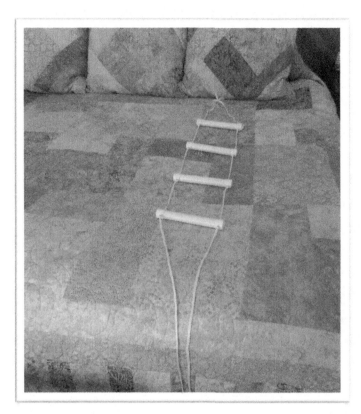

Bed Ladder

Today, there are what look like the rope ladders of yesteryear, but they serve a different purpose. Tie one end to a leg of the bed and then lay the ladder along the bed. Use the ladder to help you get up or down while in bed.

Jane has three rope ladders on her bed. Two help her get into and out of her bed as they are oriented across the bed. The other one helps her move up and down.

The rope ladders may be folded into a small space and taken with you when you travel. They are easy to install and remove from almost any bed.

Search the Internet for "bed rope ladder." You will find many to choose from. We purchased ours from Amazon.com.

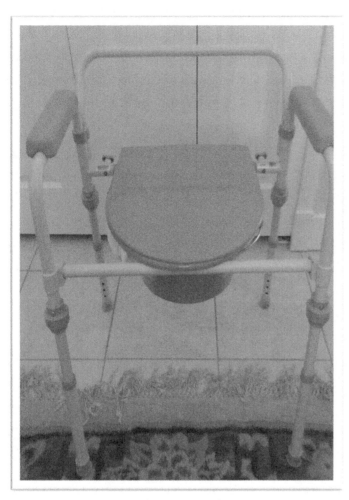

Bedside Commode

Bedside Commode

Waking up in the middle of the night with the need to "go" can be a challenge for someone with Parkinson's disease. Given that PD is often "life in slow motion," the time it takes from recognizing an urge until getting to a toilet down the hall may be too long. A simple solution is to use a bedside commode. Purchase locally or on-line. Purchase some waterproof bags and tie them tightly in the morning and dispose of them. Alternatively, use the commode container and pour the contents into a toilet and then clean the container with fresh water. Make sure the bedside commode has a lid and that the lid is secure when the commode is not in use. Failure to do so will result in a urine smell permeating the home. You may not notice the smell, but your guests will!

Waterproof Pad

Accidents do happen. Make sure the mattress has a waterproof pad. Urinary incontinence can be an issue in the later stages of PD. We will discuss ways to deal with it in Chapter 14.

CHAPTER 12 – The Kitchen

The kitchen is the second most dangerous place in the home. Sharp knives, pots of boiling water, hot ovens, etc., contribute to a lot of home kitchen accidents. Add the physical limitations that come with PD, and the risk goes up.

Jane no longer prepares meals. We decided that the kitchen was too dangerous a place for her to be during meal preparation. I now do the grocery shopping and meal preparation.

Occasionally, Jane will help with preparing food for cooking. She sits at the dining room table and does the work there. It may be cutting the ends off green beans or preparing strawberries. With a cutting board, a few dishes, and a sharp knife, she gets the satisfaction of participating in meal preparation. When Jane's dexterity is limited, she does not participate.

More than half of those with PD are men. Since women are frequently the family cook, kitchen activity can proceed as usual regardless of the Parkinson's diagnosis.

If you are a man, and a caregiver like me, then it is time for you to learn how to cook, if you do not already know how. For your culinary education, there are books, DVDs, and on-line courses. You may be able to find a cooking class nearby through a continuing education program. Get with it!

Healthy eating is important for everyone. Do not settle on what we used to call "TV dinners" as your main fare or bring home fast food every night to your loved one. Take the time to learn healthy meal planning, healthy grocery shopping, and food preparation. It will pay dividends to both of you.

I took the time to learn how to cook. I enjoy it.

I prefer doing my own grocery shopping.

There is always an array of fresh fruit in the house.

Every meal includes vegetables with a main dish such as fish or lean meat.

As the PWP becomes less mobile, it is all too easy to continue to eat more food than needed, with the result of putting on pounds. Gaining weight is not good. It exaggerates the challenge of movement for someone with PD, especially getting up and down from a seated position or getting into or out of an automobile. We are working with a nutritionist at our Parkinson's Center of Excellence. She is helping Jane fine-tune what, and how much she eats, with the objective of shaving off a few pounds while ensuring a balanced diet. Adding a nutritionist to your support staff may be a good move as well!

CHAPTER 13 – Personal

This is Jane's chapter. She wants to share with you some of the tricks she has come up with to make living at home easier for her. Jane, take it away!

Clothing

I have found that loose clothing works best for me. I like wide pant legs so that I can put on trousers when I have on shoes. Button-down-front blouses make dressing and undressing easy for me. I like my pants to have elastic in the waist or drawstrings.

Shoes

No shoelaces. Velcro ties are perfect. No sandals or flip-flops. I like snug fitting shoes as they help me with balance and with walking.

Fanny Pack

I use a fanny pack in the house, and not just when I go out. In it I carry my smartphone, pills as needed and other personal items.

Computer

Ed covered the computer in Chapter 6. I want to emphasize the importance to me of a large external monitor and external keyboard and mouse since I have Parkinson's-induced vision problems. Ed set my computer up so that everything displayed on the external monitor is large. Get someone to do that for you if you do not know how to do it yourself.

Housekeeper

I arranged a housekeeper to come to the home once a week, for four hours. She cleans the home, does the laundry, does dishes as needed, changes the beds and so forth. While she is here Ed feels free to do something outside the home without worrying about me. It has been a win-win situation.

Companion

I found a woman to serve as my companion when Ed needs to get away for a few hours. She helps me with office tasks, takes me to get my hair and nails done, and we often go out to lunch for a little girl talk! She does not provide any medical support. She is strictly a companion. There are services that can provide such a person for you.

Smartphone

I carry my smartphone wherever I go, inside or outside the home. It is usually in my fanny pack. That way, if I need help, it is just a phone call away. Ed carries his smartphone with him all the time. If we need to communicate with one another when we are not close by, we have our phones to do so.

I purchased several chargers for my phone and have located them at various places in the home. There is one in the bedroom, one in my office, and one next to the dining room table. That allows me to recharge the phone easily and have my phone nearby while doing so.

Kitchen

In chapter 12, you learned that Ed does the meal preparation. He tells me to stay out of his kitchen! However, I do venture into that space when he is not around: to get something out of the refrigerator or open a cabinet to retrieve some flatware or a dish or two. Ed puts things I might need from the refrigerator on low shelves for easy access. The same is true for dishes; some are stored in cabinets I can easily access.

CHAPTER 14 – Urinary Incontinence

This is Ed. I am back at the keyboard. Jane decided to resume the supervisory and consulting role!

When we first laid out our book, we did not include a chapter on urinary incontinence. We thought the subject too personal. Most people do not want to share that they are incontinent with their closest friends, let alone broadcast it in a book. Although the issue has impacted both of our lives, we have learned how to cope. Most recently, Jane experienced a breakthrough that has helped both of us. We decided that we would bare it all, with the hope that others might benefit from what we have learned.

Jane's incontinence did not come on suddenly. At first, she would occasionally not make it to the bathroom in time. The urge would come, but her Parkinson's disease would not allow her to move quickly enough. She discussed it with her primary care physician. He referred her to a urologist.

Her urologist was great. She did a thorough evaluation, including a minimally invasive investigation of the bladder. A fiber optic probe was inserted into the bladder so she could observe bladder function. She asked me to participate in the test. My job was to turn Jane's deep brain stimulators on and off so the urologist could evaluate Jane's bladder muscle performance with and without the DBS devices active to see if they might be contributing to the incontinence. Conclusion: they were not.

Jane's urologist prescribed a drug that has been widely used for many years for children who have bedwetting problems. The drug worked great. Problem solved, at least for a few years.

Unfortunately, after a few years, the problem came back, especially at night. More visits to a urologist. This time a surgeon. He concluded that there was nothing that could be done surgically or with medicine. Recommendation, incontinence pads.

We discussed an internal catheter with Jane's urologist. He discouraged it. The risk of urinary tract infection is too high. Safer to use the panties and pads.

For several years, Jane has been wearing incontinence panties and pads. During the day, she can visit the toilet frequently, which reduces the number of panties and pads needed. Nighttime has been a challenge. She has had to wear multiple pads with the panties and even then, about once a week there would be an overflow, urine-soaked bed linens, and dismay. The bed would have to be stripped and bedding replaced. The soiled sheets would go directly to the washer for cleaning. Sometimes this would happen in the middle of the night. Sometimes Jane would not discover it until the morning. We thought this was going to be a permanent way of life for us.

If Jane were a man, the solution would have been simple. External catheters are readily available. Do an Internet search for "male external catheters." There are many choices. The following is a description from Wikipedia.

Condom catheters, also known as male external catheters, are made of silicone or latex (depending on the brand/manufacturer) and cover the penis just like a condom but with an opening at the end to allow the connection to the urine bag. The sheath is worn over the penis and looks like a condom (hence the name). It stays in place by use of an adhesive, which can either be built into the sheath or come as a separate adhesive liner. The urine gets funneled away from the body, always keeping the skin dry. The urine runs into a urine bag that is attached at the bottom of the external catheter. During the day, a drainable leg bag can be used, and at night it is recommended to use a large-capacity bedside drainage bag. Male external catheters are designed to be worn 24/7 and changed daily. They can be used by men with both light and severe incontinence. Male external catheters come in several sizes and lengths to accommodate anatomical variation.

For a woman, the interconnection of an external catheter to the body is more challenging.

Jane recently learned about an external catheter that works perfectly for her female anatomy. It is called PureWick™. It consists of a replaceable pad that fits between her legs that connects via a flexible hose to a vacuum pump/container that she puts on the floor next to her bed. She puts the pad in place when she gets into bed for the night. The vacuum is slight. It can hardly be felt. Urine is vacuumed away and deposited into the container. The container is emptied in the morning and the container and tubing cleaned.

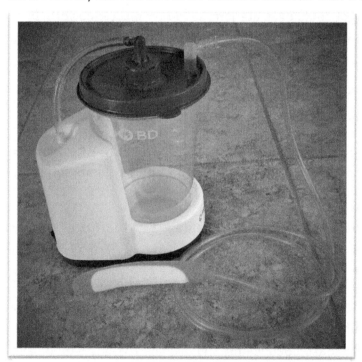

PureWick External Female Catheter

Do an Internet search for "female external catheter" or "PureWick™."

https://www.purewickathome.com/

Gone are soiled linens, the need to wear bulky panties and pads at night, and the middle of the night bedding changes, along with the dismay experienced by both of us.

CHAPTER 15 - Keeping the Caregiver Healthy

Here is some startling data. According to experts, on average, 30% of caregivers die before the person they are taking care of passes. For caregivers over the age of 70, that number grows to 70%! Do an Internet search for "Why do caregivers die first?"

The medical community has a term for it. They call it "caregiver syndrome." Reported symptoms include the following.

- Anxiety, depression, irritability
- Feeling tired and run down
- Difficulty sleeping
- Overreacting to minor nuisances
- New or worsening health problems

For the good of the caregiver, and the person with Parkinson's disease, these issues must be addressed, and as early as possible.

In our case, if I die, or become unable to function as Jane's caregiver, she will immediately need to move to an assisted living facility or a nursing home. This is likely true for many Parkinson's couples.

In this chapter you will learn about what we do, or try to do, to ensure the best caregiver health possible.

Separate Bedroom

Ten years ago, it became evident to me that I was in a state of constant brain fog. It was as if my body and mind did what needed to be done, but my soul was just a passenger, traveling along with my body, observing everyday life. It was lowering my quality of life. Time to see my doctor.

My doctor knew Jane had Parkinson's disease as he was also her doctor. He quickly zeroed in on my sleep, and our sleeping arrangements. He concluded that although I spent eight hours in bed each night, I was not getting restful sleep. He knew that Jane suffered from REM (rapid eye movement) sleep disorder, which is a common Parkinson's symptom. His recommendation: sleep in separate bedrooms.

I moved into our guest bedroom. Within a few days my condition improved. In a week, I was cured!

We have slept in separate bedrooms ever since, except for when we travel.

When we travel, I carry a battery operated noise maker. It can produce the sound of rain, ocean waves breaking on the beach, or white noise. I find a background sound helps drown out the noise Jane makes when her sleep disorder kicks-in.

Need for Frequent Time Away

The professionals recommend caregivers have a day a week to themselves, a long weekend once a month and a week away once a quarter. My experience is that few caregivers comply.

Since Jane has a companion who visits her several times a week, I now have an opportunity to lunch with friends, participate in sports, attend lectures, or just take a long walk in the park. The companion provides value to both of us.

Getting away for a longer period is challenging. It has proven difficult for us to find someone to stay with Jane for days or weeks at a time. You may be faced with the same issue. Try your best to surmount the problem. Reach out to friends and family. If you can afford it, pay for short-term, live-in help. Look at the big picture. Paying for help now may prove far less expensive than paying for resident care well before it would otherwise be needed.

My favorite caregiver break is a short trip on a cruise ship. See chapter 23 for details.

Hobbies

When you cannot get away for a caregiver break, having a hobby at home can reduce stress. In my case, I enjoy building things. Do what you enjoy. The important thing is to have a hobby to afford you an occasional escape from your daily responsibilities as a caregiver, even if only for an hour or two.

Music

I find that putting on a good set of headphones to listen to music provides a few minutes isolation from my caregiver responsibilities, yet I am readily available to assist Jane if needed. I connect my noise-cancelling headphones to my smartphone. The music is streamed via an App such as Sirius XM Radio™ or Pandora™. There are plenty of music apps available, both paid and free. Those are the two I use. The advantage of my using my smartphone is that Jane can call my mobile number if she needs me. The music is interrupted, and we speak.

CHAPTER 16 - Do not Fall—Use an Assist Device

I am beginning this chapter with a warning. A PWP needs to work with a medical professional when choosing an assist device. You want a device that will help maintain your mobility while reducing your chance of falling. Mobility problems vary from one Parkinson's person to another. What works for Jane may not be good for you.

When should someone with Parkinson's disease begin using an assist device? The answer is, before a fall. Better to begin using a device early than after it is too late.

None of us wants to use a cane or walker. It is an admission that we are going through irreversible changes in our life. What to do? Accept it and move on.

Community Loaner Program

You might be tempted to rush out and purchase something as soon as it becomes evident the time has come to use an assist device. Before you do, check out some alternatives.

Check your local senior center or community service organization. They may have canes, walkers, and manual wheelchairs available for short- or long-term loan, or for purchase.

Even if you want to purchase new, you may want to try out alternatives by borrowing before buying.

The civic center in our community has dozens of mobility devices available of many different types. They receive so many device donations every year, that they run out of storage. They are more than happy to make a loan!

Thrift stores are another source of canes, walkers, and wheelchairs. You might even be lucky and find an electric scooter or electric wheelchair!

Canes

In Chapter 7, I described Jane's ambulator. It is a cane with a horizontal rod located near floor level. Jane uses it as a triggering device to get her feet moving when they feel like they are glued to the floor. She has never used the cane to help her with balance, or to keep her from falling.

Because we have no other experience using a cane, this is the limit of our cane discussion.

Walkers

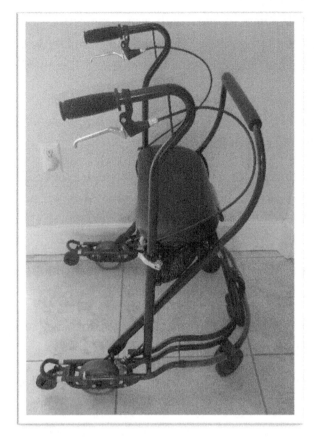

U-Step Walker

Earlier, I mentioned that Jane fell twice, requiring visits to the hospital. These were not her only falls. She has had several others, but fortunately has not been hurt. Each time she visited her neurologist, he would ask if she had fallen since he had last seen her. When she reported a recent fall, he recommended she use a walker. His choice was the Parkinson's U-Step walker.

To learn more about the U-Step walker, go to:

https://www.ustep.com/

or search the Internet for "Parkinson's U-Step Walker."

The U-Step walker has brakes that work opposite from a bicycle. These brakes are normally engaged. Squeeze the brake handles and the brakes release. The user releases the brakes only when movement is desired.

The U-Step walker has a seat. When Jane got tired, she could turn around and sit down. She seldom needed the seat.

Jane did not use the U-Step for long. The problem for her was its weight and bulk. She was still driving, and often out on her own. Lifting the 22-pound walker into the trunk of her car proved too difficult.

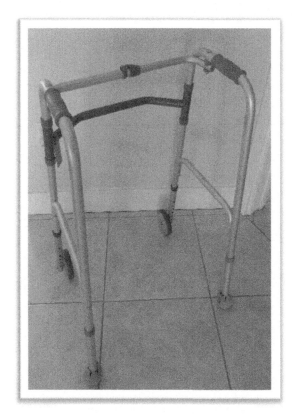

Jane decided to try a lightweight aluminum walker. There are many to choose from. Local drug stores sell them. Walmart sells them. They are readily available online. Some sell for less than thirty dollars. They fold up easily. Many weigh less than ten pounds. After the rubber feet in the back legs of the walker wore through, Jane had me buy two tennis balls into which I cut slits with a hacksaw. The tennis balls replaced the rubber feet. Today, you can purchase pre-slit tennis balls for just that purpose. Go to Amazon.com and search for "pre-slit tennis balls for walkers."

Lightweight Aluminum Walker

The lightweight aluminum walker worked well for Jane for several years, but eventually she had difficulty walking more than a hundred feet, mostly because her freezing episodes slowed her down. She would use her triggering device combined with the walker to get her moving while the walker provided stability. This was not optimal. We then realized it was time for a scooter, which I will elaborate on in the next chapter.

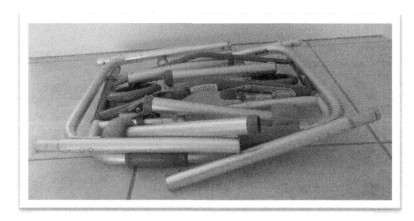

When we travel, Jane gets around with a wheelchair, but in a hotel room she still needs her walker. We had to figure out how to carry the walker along with suitcases and the other supplies needed when she is away from home. Our solution was the purchase of a lightweight aluminum walker that could be quickly disassembled and put into a suitcase and then easily reassembled when needed.

Collapsible Aluminum Walker

Do an Internet search for "collapsible aluminum walker." We found ours on Amazon.com.

CHAPTER 17 - Increasing Your Mobility

Jane began her enhanced mobility experience by using scooters that were available at our local grocery store. Our observation is that most grocery stores and many of the big-box stores have them. They are a good way for you to get some scooter experience while making your shopping easier.

Our next scooter experience was on a cruise ship. We rented one. After several cruises and theme parks with rental scooters, we decided it was time for Jane to have one of her own. It took several years before we found the scooter that was ideal for us. I mention us, because the choice of a scooter (and a mobility device in general) impacts the lives of both the PWP and the caregiver.

We quickly discovered that our automobile, which was a sedan, was not the right choice since we now traveled with a scooter. We could have added a hitch to the car and then had an apparatus installed that would allow us to carry the scooter behind the car. After some investigation, we decided not to do that. Instead, we sold the car and purchased a minivan.

Do an Internet search for "mobility scooter carriers" if you are interested in adding one to your car. There are manual and electric versions. The scooter is driven onto the carrier and then the carrier is raised into the travel position, either electrically or manually. The advantage is that there is no need to disassemble the scooter or do any lifting. The disadvantage is that the scooter is out in the weather. Of course, a cover could be purchased and installed to protect it.

The scooter worked well for Jane for several years. Eventually she found that if she got off the scooter and sat in a chair for an hour or two, she had difficulty getting up and back onto the scooter without help from others. This was an issue for us, especially when we were at a restaurant. One evening, we had to enlist help from the wait staff to pick Jane up from her chair and deposit her onto her scooter. Time for a new plan. We sold the scooter and purchased a power wheelchair. That way, she could remain in her wheelchair and not have to make the transition to a restaurant chair and back. That is her status today.

We added manual wheelchairs to our collection of mobility devices at the same time we purchased the electrically powered wheelchair.

We now have four wheelchairs. Two are powered and two are manual. Why so many? Time to explain.

We have a lightweight powered wheelchair that stays in the back of our minivan. In the house, Jane has a different powered wheelchair for use around the house. We have a small manual chair that Jane takes when she goes out with friends in their vehicle. We have a larger manual chair with large wheels that stays in the house. Jane gets exercise by moving herself around the home using arm-power!

Do not constrain yourself to having only one mobility aid if more will make your life easier and you can afford the extra expense.

Device Weight – A Major Consideration

We learned early in our scooter experience that weight is an important consideration. If it is difficult for either the PWP or the caregiver to move a mobility device into or out of an automobile, then they both become reluctant to leave home unless necessary. Fortunately, scooters, manual wheelchairs, and power wheelchairs are all available in lightweight versions. In the remainder of this chapter, we will share our initial experience with a heavy device, and then the purchase that met our weight goal.

Scooters

The scooters we rented looked like a model called the Spitfire Scout. Do an Internet search for "Spitfire Scout 4-wheel mobility scooter." You will find that exact model as well as similar devices.

When we decided to buy our own, we went to a local scooter store to arrange the purchase. Wow, did we get an education!

Jane asked her doctor for a letter of authorization for scooter purchase so that some of the cost would be covered by her health insurance. She presented that to the scooter store. "No problem," they said, and that the cost would be $2,400 with some of that covered by Medicare. Fortunately, we had done our homework. We knew we could purchase the exact same scooter online for $700, with shipping included. "Why the additional cost?", we asked. The answer was that Medicare required the scooter store to deliver the device to our home, unpack it, assemble it, and then provide instruction on its use. Since the scooter was to be purchased from their store, the price was retail,

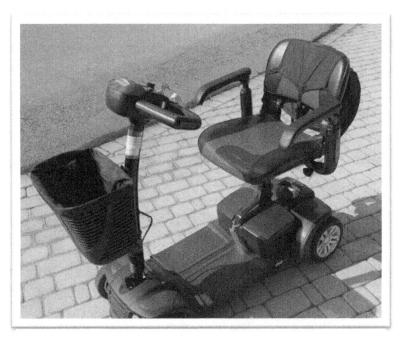

Jane's Red Spitfire Mobility Scooter

which was higher than the online price. Jane asked what her out of pocket cost would be after the Medicare reimbursement. The answer was that our cost would be more than it would cost us to purchase directly from an online seller. We left the store and later that day ordered online. In a few days, the scooter arrived. I quickly unpacked and assembled it, and moments later, Jane was scooting around the neighborhood!

Jane's Red Spitfire weighed over 100 lbs. I could disassemble it into 4 pieces in a few minutes, without the need for tools. I would take it apart and put the pieces into the back of our sedan. Unfortunately, the parts were not light. The battery pack was over 30 pounds. Leaning over the trunk of the car to put in or take out 30 pounds was not something my back would tolerate. When we sold the car and bought a minivan, the need to lean over was less significant, but the need for lifting heavy items did not go away.

I found that disassembling and reassembling the Spitfire was not easy, especially in bad weather. I had to bend down to street level to conduct the process. All too often, I got my clothes dirty.

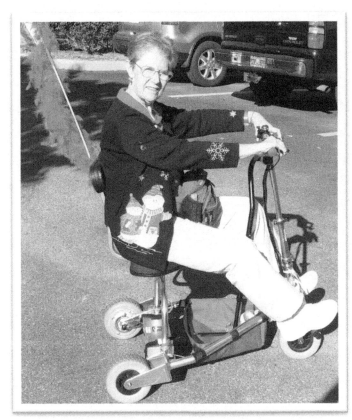

Jane on her TravelScoot

A few years later, while on a trip, I saw someone driving an all-aluminum scooter that was lightweight. I asked the owner what it was. She told me it was a TravelScoot™. When I got home, I went online and checked it out. I liked what I saw. Including the battery, the scooter weighs only 35-pounds. It could be quickly folded into a compact package and put into the trunk of a car. Unfolding looked easy as well. I watched the videos that were online. I was impressed.

If you would like to learn more about the TravelScoot™, go to:

https://www.travelscootusa.com

When driving a TravelScoot™, the user must have the hand strength and the cognitive ability to be able to operate the two manual brakes. The brakes work just like a bicycle. When going down a hill, if one lets off on the power, the scooter does not stop. One must manually apply the brakes. For that reason, a TravelScoot™ may not be a good choice for everyone with Parkinson's disease. For Jane, it proved to be perfect.

We sold the Red Spitfire and purchased a TravelScoot™.

I found that I could easily put the TravelScoot™ into the back of our minivan. I would lift the front wheel over the rear bumper, then rotate the scooter up and into the van. Since the front wheel was resting on the vehicle, I only needed to lift half of the weight, about 18-pounds. Easy!

Today, if you do an Internet search for "lightweight mobility scooters" you will find many alternatives. My recent search suggests the TravelScoot™ still holds the low-weight record, although others come close. Make sure when you do your scooter evaluation that the stated weight includes the batteries. Many scooters now use lithium-ion batteries which are lightweight and have long-life. Some manufacturers still use sealed lead-acid batteries which are substantially heavier and have limited life. You want to know the total weight of the scooter, batteries included.

One concern I had with a scooter in the back of our van was what would happen if we were in an automobile accident. Would the scooter fly forward and decapitate us? My solution was to make a mounting platform. I include what I did not as specific instructions, but to give you an idea of how I addressed the issue.

I did not want to drill holes into our van. I took a 36 inch x 18 inch x ½ inch piece of particle board and screwed and glued a wood frame into it that holds the scooter's wheels. Rings were attached to wooden parts that were screwed

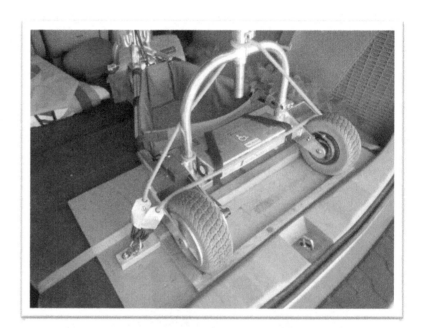

TravelScoot™ Mounting Platform

and glued firmly into the particle board. A ratcheting strap was added that firmly holds the assembly to the folded-down rear seat. Two elastic straps hold the scooter in place.

Powered Wheelchairs

When it was time to purchase a power wheelchair we knew to look for something lightweight. I needed to be able to easily get the chair into and out of our minivan without straining my back.

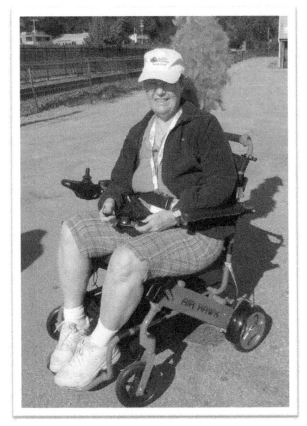

Jane's Lightweight Power Wheelchair

Do an Internet search for "power wheelchair." You will find that there are many different ones available.

Our search found a chair that weighed 41 pounds without batteries. It is called the Air Hawk. Each lithium-ion battery added five pounds. We elected to purchase two batteries. There are mounts for both. One is active and the other a spare. The batteries can be swapped in seconds. With two batteries, we have a range of 20 miles! We go many days between charging.

Our chair will fold up and can fit between the passenger seat and the seat behind it. I suspect it would fit in some cars. Since we have a van, I prefer to put it in the back, with no need to fold and unfold.

I used the same techniques to get the chair in and out of our van as I did with the scooter. I put the front wheels over the rear bumper and then lift the chair into place. That way, with both batteries installed, I only need to lift 25 pounds. I do the reverse when removing the chair. This has worked great.

Once the chair is in the van and tied down, I fold the upright chair seat down so my view out the rear-view mirror is not obstructed.

I modified the mounting platform that I had made for Jane's scooter to fit the power wheelchair.

One issue I had was that the front wheels are not driven, and they readily rotated the wrong way the first time I tried to get the chair into the van. The solution was simple. I made a few wooden stops which I can put in the wheels to lock them in place. Your chair may be different. I include my solution so that you might produce a fix for your chair if you encounter a similar problem.

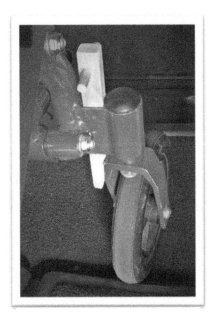

Wooden Wheel Lock Plug

Jane loves her lightweight power wheelchair. She did find it uncomfortable for use in the home where she will often be seated for hours at a time. She tried different cushions but did not find anything that worked. She also felt the chair's rear-wheel drive could not maneuver in tight places to her satisfaction.

We purchased a front wheel drive power wheelchair with a well-padded seat, just for her use in our home. We went to a local mobility store to try out different chairs. The store brought the candidate chair to our home for Jane's pre-purchase evaluation. I did remove one arm rest to provide better clearance for her when she needs to maneuver in tight places. This has saved a few door frames!

Dress up your Mobility Device for Safety

We recommend a flag staff for your scooter or wheelchair. Look at the picture of Jane driving the TravelScoot and her power wheelchair. I mounted a 36-inch fiberglass rod to both the scooter and the wheelchair. The fiberglass rod is decorated with a red boa. At the top is a flag. Since we live in the USA, the flag is the stars and stripes!

You can buy a flag staff at a bicycle shop or purchase one online. Search for "bicycle flagpole."

Jane gets stopped by people who want to tell her how colorful her boa and flag are. She explains that they are there for safety. When she is traversing parking lots, she is more easily seen by drivers with her red boa flying in the wind!

We have found having the boa/flag combination helps when Jane is trying to get into an elevator when there is a crowd of people trying to do the same. People may not see someone in a wheelchair as their lines-of-sight are usually horizontal and not downward. They cannot miss Jane's red boa!

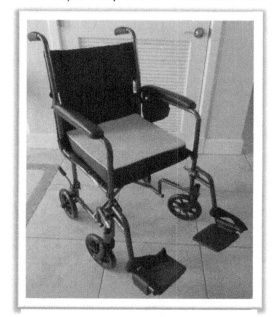

Lightweight Transport Wheelchair

Manual Wheelchairs

A lightweight transport wheelchair has proved to be an excellent investment. Ours weighs 19 pounds. It is easily put into the trunk of a car or behind the passenger seat. It must, of course, be pushed as it has no motor. The footrests are easily removed and replaced.

Jane purchased a cushion for the chair for increased comfort when sitting for long periods.

The chair can be folded or unfolded in a few seconds.

We use this chair when we visit friends. Jane's power chair is wider and sometimes it is a challenge to get into and or around some homes. This chair has never let us down.

When Jane goes out with her lady friends, this is the chair they take.

We live in a golf cart community. People use their golf carts for local transportation as well as when playing golf.

Jane loves our golf cart. It is a way for her to get fresh air. She calls it her convertible, although the top does not come down. When we considered purchasing a cart, the first thing we considered was how to take a wheelchair with us. There was no way to carry her power chair. A quick check confirmed her lightweight transport chair would fit perfectly on the back of the cart, where two golf bags normally go. The straps that normally hold the golf bags worked perfectly to hold her chair.

When we get to our destination, it takes just a few seconds for me to remove and unfold the chair. There are few hills where we live, so pushing the chair takes little effort. It is good exercise for me!

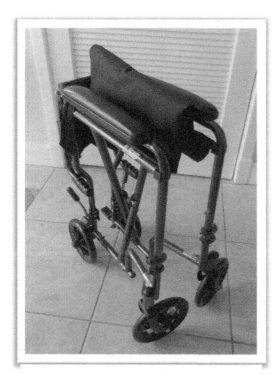

Transport Wheelchair Folded

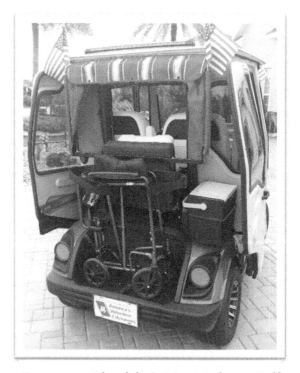

Transport Wheelchair Mounted to a Golf Cart

CHAPTER 18 – Lift Assist

In our community, there is a special phone number to call if you need assistance getting up and there is no one immediately available to help you. The service is called "lift assist." Call that number and some strong young guys and gals come to the home to get you up. They are with the fire department. They do not come with their siren blazing but they do come in their big fire engine. We keep the lift assist phone number in our smartphones and a copy of the number is taped to the refrigerator for ready access if someone other than Jane or I need to make the call. I have used this service several times, most recently when Jane slipped out of her wheelchair onto the carpet in front of the sofa. It was a transfer gone bad! I will not try to pick Jane up as I cannot risk a back injury. The responders from the fire company came, and when I opened the door they asked, "Where is Jane?". She is on a first name basis with these fine folks.

CHAPTER 19 - Off to the Hospital

A few years ago, Jane suffered a fall. She was in the hospital for three days, and then discharged to a nursing home for in-patient rehabilitation. I will discuss the rehabilitation experience in the next chapter.

Jane's hospital experience was not positive. Some of the blame is ours. We did not arrive prepared. At the time, we did not know how to prepare. Now we do.

In this chapter, you will learn how to prepare both of you for a hospital visit and what to do once there. The visit may be planned or unexpected. The key to a good visit is to have a "to-go" kit, ready for the caregiver or the PWP to scoop up as you head out, be it by your own car or by ambulance.

To-Go Kit

Some great news. The "to-go" kit is easy to prepare. The hard work has already been done for you. The kit you need is called "Aware in Care" and is available from the Parkinson's Foundation. Do an Internet search for "Parkinson's Hospital Kit - Parkinson's Foundation" or enter the following into your browser:

https://www.parkinson.org/Living-with-Parkinsons/Resources-and-Support/Hospital-Kit

The above site offers three options: download free printable resources; order a free Aware in Care packet; or order a complete Aware in Care Kit that is free but requires payment of a small shipping charge. The last option includes a zippered pouch that contains almost all the information you will need to take with you to the hospital.

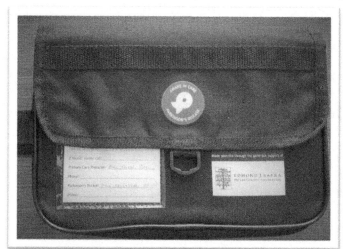

Jane's Aware in Care Hospital Bag

The site includes a link to download a copy of a hospitalization letter that we recommend you fill out and have signed by your neurologist. Put that letter in your kit.

When you get your kit, fill in the information recommended. The kit provides the most value for you only if you personalize it.

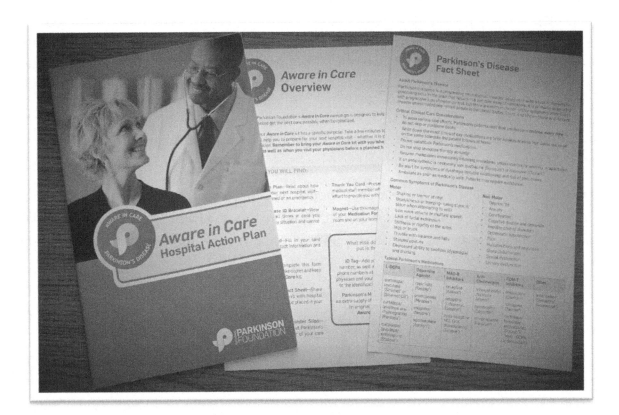

Examples of Aware in Care Bag Contents

Advance Directives

A hospital admission staff will ask about certain legal documents and will ask for copies. The name of the documents may differ from state to state.

A Combination Living Will and Designation of a Health Care Surrogate is the name used in Florida.

Regardless of the name, you need to identify the patient's legal representative to the hospital in the event the PWP is unable to make decisions for himself/herself. In addition, the patient needs to define what the hospital staff is to do in an end-of-life situation.

We suggest you contact an attorney to have the appropriate documents prepared.

Put copies of the advanced directives in your "to-go" kit.

You Need an Advocate

Upon admittance to a hospital, you will need an advocate. Your caregiver is the logical person.

The first thing the advocate should do is make sure the hospital staff reads everything in the "to-go" kit. Ask them to sign that they have read and understand everything. The advocate should closely supervise the PWP's care, including making sure drugs are correct and taken on time. If care is not adequate, the advocate needs to take concerns up the management chain until there is resolution. Be pleasant but firm.

The advocate needs to be with the PWP as much of the day and night as possible. It is a demanding but rewarding job.

CHAPTER 20 - Where to Go if You Need Rehabilitation

In chapter 19, I said that Jane had once fallen, was in a hospital for three days, and then discharged to a nursing home for inpatient rehabilitation. As with the hospital stay, this was not a positive experience for either of us. Some of the blame was ours. We did not know the difference between a skilled nursing facility and a rehabilitation hospital. In fact, we did not know rehabilitation hospitals existed.

Three days passed and Jane had not received any treatment. She spent most of her day in bed, watching TV. She told me that her drugs were not administered on time.

I asked for a meeting with the managing director and the on-site physician. I explained to the managing director that failure to prepare a written treatment plan within two days of admittance was a violation of her corporation's policy. If she did not correct it immediately, I would go as high as necessary within her company to get the issue resolved.

The on-site physician said that he had evaluated Jane and found her mentally and physically capable of taking her drugs herself. Problem solved.

Within hours, there was a written care plan in-place and physical therapy began.

Jane received one hour of therapy a day. I told the staff that was inadequate. They told me that it was the standard for a skilled nursing facility. The facility did allow me to give Jane additional physical therapy. They would not allow me to bring in an outside professional.

A week later, Jane was discharged. We did not go directly home. Our Parkinson's support group met later that morning. We went to it. The topic was rehabilitation hospitals!

We learned that there was a hospital 50 miles from us that specialized in rehabilitation. It was not a skilled nursing facility. The presenter told the audience that a patient there receives at least three hours of physical therapy a day, other aggressive programs to prepare them to return home, and social interaction. He said that admittance to his hospital did not require a previous hospital stay, only an evaluation from his medical staff.

We wish we had known about rehabilitation hospitals two weeks earlier. That is where Jane should have gone. The outcome would have been better. Yes, it was an hour's drive from where we lived, but sometimes one must travel to get an optimal outcome.

Let me provide you some further education about rehabilitation alternatives.

Inpatient Rehabilitation Alternatives

The following definitions are worth understanding.

1. *By definition, a skilled nursing facility is a healthcare institution that has at least one full-time registered nurse (many facilities have much more than this on staff at any given time) as well as a doctor, provides nursing care 24 hours a day, and has a place to store and dispense medication. They may have on-site physical therapists, or they may have those people come in as needed.*

2. *Rehabilitation hospitals, also referred to as inpatient rehabilitation hospitals, focus on the rehabilitation of patients with various neurological, musculoskeletal, orthopedic, and other medical conditions following stabilization of their acute medical issues. The industry mostly consists of independent hospitals that operate these facilities within acute care hospitals. There are also inpatient rehabilitation hospitals that offer this service in a hospital-like setting but separate from acute care facilities. Most inpatient rehabilitation facilities are located within hospitals.*

The American Hospital Association website provides a detailed comparison of skilled nursing facilities and inpatient rehabilitation facilities. It is worth reading. Go to:

https://www.aha.org/

Search the site for "fact sheet inpatient rehabilitation facilities." Click on the first result. You will find a link to a PDF file. Click on it. The following is from that file:

Medicare Requirements for Inpatient Rehabilitation Facility (IRF) vs. Skilled Nursing Facility (SNF)	IRFs	SNFs
Physician approval of preadmission screen and admission	Yes	No
Patient requires resource-intensive inpatient care	Yes	No
Close medical supervision by a physician with specialized training	Yes	No
Physician-coordinated multidisciplinary team, including medical plan of care, 24-hour registered nurse care and therapy	Yes	No
3 hours of intensive therapy; 5 days per week	Yes	No
Discharge rate to community*	76.0%	40.0%
Potentially-avoidable rehospitalization during stay*	2.6%	10.9%
Potentially-avoidable rehospitalization during 30 days after discharge*	4.7%	6.1%

Note the three hours of intensive therapy, five days a week for an inpatient rehabilitation facility.

Locating an Inpatient Rehabilitation Hospital

Do an Internet search for "rehabilitation hospitals *your state or city*" or try "rehabilitation hospitals near me."

Check the website for each place you find. Make sure they are a rehabilitation hospital and not a skilled nursing facility. See how much physical therapy they provide each day. Look for three hours or more.

CHAPTER 21 – Driving

Handicap Parking Permit

Once Jane's freezing of gait became significant, her primary care physician recommended she get a handicap parking permit. He filled out paperwork which she submitted to the motor vehicle department. Check with your local motor vehicle department to find out how you obtain yours.

A handicap parking permit is assigned to the person and not to a vehicle.

Jane carries her permit with her if she is going to be riding in a vehicle other than ours.

I never use Jane's permit for myself as I am not handicapped. I park in a non-handicap space if I am alone or if she is with me but not getting out.

Getting Into and Out of the Car

It can take Jane several minutes to get into or out of our car. She has learned how to grab onto handholds to help her maneuver. A device she finds useful is a "vehicle support handle." They can be purchased at Walmart, a drug store, or online. The handle is inserted into the door latch which gives her another place to hold on to. Once in the car, she makes sure the handle has been removed and stored. Otherwise, attempting to close the door might damage the handle or the car!

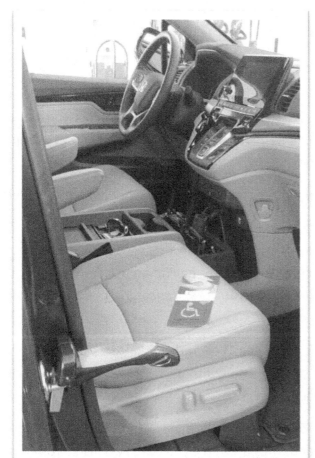

Vehicle Support Handle Inserted into the Door Latch

Handicap Parking Permit on the Seat Ready to be Hung from the Rear-View Mirror

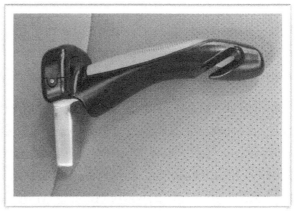

Vehicle Support Handle

Safety Features of Newer Automobiles

Two years ago, we purchased a new Honda Odyssey minivan. It was one of the more expensive models. We wanted a vehicle with advanced safety features. Many new cars available now (2022 model year) have these features. Examples include lane departure warning, lane-keeping assist, adaptive cruise control, emergency braking, blind-spot monitoring, rear cross-traffic alert, and more.

Some features are active all the time. Others must be activated by the driver each time the car is started. In my case, two that I want engaged are lane-keeping assist and adaptive cruise control with emergency braking. I turn them on each time I drive the car. I activate the adaptive cruise control once up to the speed desired.

If you have Parkinson's disease and are still driving, consider purchasing an automobile with the above features. Learn how to use the devices and activate them wherever possible. It could make the difference between a safe trip and an accident.

Should You Be Driving?

Most people will agree that driving an automobile is a multi-task activity. One must constantly observe the road and vehicles nearby, make instantaneous assessment of the need to change direction, brake or accelerate, be aware of people nearby, navigate, etc.

An early symptom of Parkinson's disease is the inability to multi-task. Given that fact, ask yourself if you should be driving!

About ten years ago, Jane announced that she no longer felt safe driving. She had a serious concern that her lack of ability to multi-task might result in her having an accident where she might hurt someone, including herself. She turned in her driver's license and got a non-driver state-issued ID.

When Jane and I give our presentation, "Ideas for Living Well with Parkinson's Disease," we discuss driving. Our recommendation is that if you want to continue to drive, do not seek the approval of your doctor, seek the approval of your lawyer!

Suppose you are in an accident, and someone is killed or seriously injured. You get sued. The case goes to court. The prosecutor gets you on the stand. They ask you if you have Parkinson's disease. You answer "yes." Next, they bring in an expert to tell the court about the problem someone with Parkinson's disease has with any activity that requires multi-tasking. Another expert appears to help the court understand that driving is multi-tasking to the extreme. Case closed. You lose. You lose not only the case, but you may also lose everything you have worked for all your life: your savings, your home, your pension.

Jane decided she did not want to put her life savings at risk, nor could she bear the emotional burden if she were to severely injure or kill someone.

We have attended support group meetings where a person with Parkinson's disease had proudly told the group that they took a motor vehicle test and passed. So, they say they are OK to drive. One question one should ask, is where on the on/off cycle of their medication they were when they took the test. They might have been safe to drive when "on" but dangerous when "off."

Men can be a problem. Giving up driving might be considered a loss of manhood to many. Guys, get over it! Do not put your caregiver, your family and friends, or others at risk because you are determined to continue to drive when your Parkinson's disease says you should not. Hang up the keys. Let someone else do the driving.

CHAPTER 22 – Flying

We have traveled extensively in the last 25 years. Parkinson's disease has not stopped us. In the next chapter, we will tell you about our favorite vacation: cruise ships. Sometimes we drive to our port of departure, but other times we fly. We have learned how someone with Parkinson's disease can best deal with the challenges of commercial flying. That is what this chapter will reveal.

Where to Sit

For short trips, we sit towards the front of the cabin to minimize the distance Jane needs to go from the plane's door to her seat. For longer trips, if flying coach class, we sit in the back, close to the restrooms.

Boarding Assistance

If you are capable of walking to your seat from the waiting area, but Parkinson's disease slows you down, take advantage of early boarding. Once the airplane lands, stay seated until others have deplaned. That will give you time to get off without feeling rushed.

Since Jane is now in an electric wheelchair, she drives her chair to the cabin entrance, and then gets to her seat with help from the crew. Airlines have special wheelchairs that navigate the aircraft's narrow aisles. They transfer her to their chair and roll her to her seat.

I leave her electric wheelchair near the cabin entrance. The luggage team takes the chair and puts it in the baggage compartment. Once the airplane has landed, they bring the chair to the cabin entrance and the boarding process is reversed.

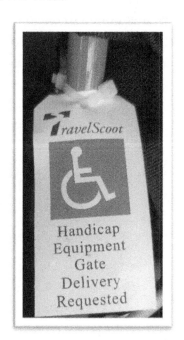

Ask the airline for a tag to put on your scooter or wheelchair. That way they know to bring it to the cabin entrance upon landing and not deliver it to a baggage carousel.

I call the airline a few days ahead of our trip to inform them we need boarding assistance. That way, they are prepared for us.

The Federal Aviation Administration (FAA) has requirements for the carrying of batteries for an electric wheelchair or electric scooter on commercial airplanes. Since requirements change, I go to the FAA website a few weeks before departure to learn the latest.

https://www.faa.gov/

I enter "electric wheelchair batteries" into the search box on the FAA website. That takes me to information for wheelchairs as well as scooters.

The airlines may require that lithium-ion batteries used in a scooter or electric wheelchair be removed and brought into the cabin for storage during the flight. As Jane's caregiver, I get that assignment. I check with the gate agent before boarding to find out what is required.

The Advantages of Flying First Class

Some of our flights have been from one coast of the country to the other. These were long flights. After a few coach class flights that proved difficult for Jane, we decided to save up and fly first class. What a difference. Her seat was always only a few feet from the cabin door. She was close to the restroom. Since the first class crew serviced fewer passengers, we found Jane received the attention she needed for restroom stops, water for taking pills, and so forth. Of course, she enjoyed flying first class, and as her caregiver I was forced to do the same!

Miraculous Recovery?

A short story. We were on a two hour domestic flight, on our way home from a long vacation. Nine people had arranged for the airline to provide them wheelchairs for boarding. Jane was one of the nine, although she had her own electric wheelchair. All of us boarded early. This flight was coach class only with unassigned seating. Upon landing, seven of the "disabled" folks jumped out of their seats and deplaned with the rest of the crowd. As we waited for deplaning assistance, we mentioned to one of the crew what we had observed. We were told the airlines have a term for it. It is called "miraculous recovery"! People game the system. By early boarding they got their choice of the best seats, and they found plenty of room for storing their personal items overhead. Sad!

CHAPTER 23 – Vacationing

We encourage people diagnosed with Parkinson's disease to get out and do their bucket list before mobility limitations make it impossible. We did exactly that. However, as the years passed, it became increasingly difficult for Jane to participate in activities requiring substantial physical exertion and fine-tuned mobility. Our solution: go cruising, not on our boat but on those piloted by others.

Cruise Ships

We have hundreds of days on cruise ships, both international and domestic. To us, it is the perfect venue for a PWP and the caregiver. What we like is that we only need to unpack and pack once; food preparation and serving is done by others; there is live as well as prerecorded entertainment; and there

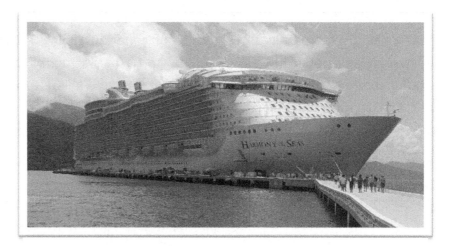

One of our Cruises in Royal Caribbean's Harmony of the Seas

are places to visit, new cultures to experience, beautiful scenery, fascinating people to meet, and long-term friendships to cultivate.

We have taken cruises as short as five days and as long as 35 days. We find 10 days ideal, although our 35 day roundtrip cruise out of Boston to Europe via Labrador, Greenland, and Iceland was so enjoyable that we did it twice, several years apart. We would love to be able to do it again!

We find cruising cost-effective. It is difficult to find another venue that includes accommodations, first-class dining, entertainment, travel, and being pampered, at the cost per person per day that is available on a large cruise ship.

Handicap Cabins

For someone with Parkinson's disease who does not need mobility assistance beyond a walker or a small manual collapsible wheelchair, a regular cabin may be adequate. The mobility aids may be brought into the cabin and stored out of the way. That is what we did in our early days of cruising. Jane did have to be careful as the bathrooms in our "regular" cabins were not always handicap friendly.

As mentioned in an earlier section of the book, Jane rented a scooter for a few cruises so that she did not have to walk the long distances encountered on large ocean-going ships. On our first cruise with a rental, a problem became apparent. We were not allowed to store a scooter or wheelchair in the hallway. It had to go into our room when not in use. The rental scooter would not fit through our cabin's doorway. We appealed to our room attendant. He arranged to store the scooter for us when we did not need it. He plugged it in overnight, so the scooter was charged and ready to go in the morning. This was a one-cruise deal. We would not be so lucky the next time. Since then, we always reserve a handicap cabin.

Different cruise lines have different standards for handicap cabins. Royal Caribbean has one type. It is large enough for a power wheelchair or scooter to turn completely around and to access the bed. Holland America has three classes of handicap cabins; a door wide enough to get a wheelchair or scooter into the room, but no further; a room large enough for wheelchair or scooter access to the side of one bed; and a room that is handicap accessible to both sides of the bed. Other cruise lines may have different standards. These are the two familiar to us. We recommend contacting the cruise line before booking to determine what type of handicap room one might need.

Booking a handicap cabin can be difficult to impossible. There are very few handicap cabins on any single ship. Those sell out quickly, often 18 months or more in advance of the sailing date. We once took a cruise simply because we did a search of a cruise line's offerings and found a cruise with an available handicap cabin. It was not our first choice of port or itinerary, but it offered us a chance to go on vacation.

Jane needs a bedside commode when she cruises. We contact the cruise line prior to the cruise to arrange one. They will provide it, so we have no need to carry one onboard.

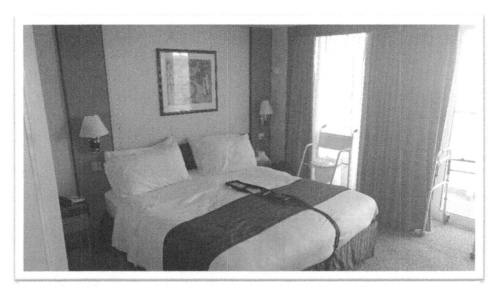

One of Our Handicap Cabins. Jane's Ladder on the Bed. Bedside Commode Next to the Bed. Collapsible Walker (assembled) to the Right. White-noise Maker on the Table Left of the Bed.

In the last few years, we have taken inland river cruises in the USA. The ships are small, typically carrying fewer than 200 passengers. By the end of a week-long cruise, you have met most everyone onboard. We have cruised the Snake and Columbia Rivers, the entire Mississippi River,

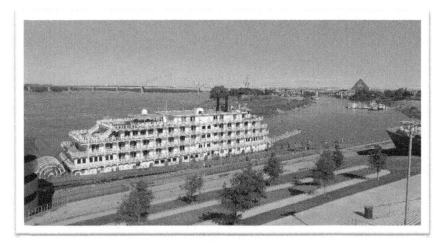

Cruising the Mississippi River on a Paddle-wheeler

and the San Juan Islands in the State of Washington. One advantage for us, as US residents, is that we are always near medical care covered by our health insurance. We have had to use it!

Insurance

We always get travel insurance. To be insured for pre-existing conditions, such as Parkinson's disease, one must purchase the insurance within a few days of making the cruise deposit. Otherwise, if a person with Parkinson's disease cancels a few days before the cruise due to a Parkinson's-related medical issue, the insurance may not cover the cancellation.

Reimbursement for our cruise deposit in the event of a medical issue is not the major reason we buy travel insurance. If one of us gets ill while on the cruise, and must be evacuated, the cost can run into the many tens of thousands of dollars. If an air-evacuation is required, cost can go beyond $100,000. That is the reason we carry trip insurance.

We often do not purchase our trip insurance from the cruise ship company. There are independent insurers that focus on travel insurance. Search the Internet for "travel insurance." Before buying, read each policy in detail. Each supplier has different benefits and restrictions. Compare the policies from the independents to that offered by the cruise company. Purchase the policy that meets your needs.

CHAPTER 24 – Parkinson's and Pets

Jane and I have enjoyed pets throughout our lives. Growing up, she had a cat, and later, a pet rabbit. My childhood included ducks, chickens, a goat, hamsters, dogs, and cats. In my adult life, I became especially fond of Siamese cats.

When Jane and I got together, 25 years ago, I had two Siamese cats: Sukiyaki and Nefertiti. Suki had lived a long life. He passed shortly thereafter. Nefertiti was young. We enjoyed her company for many years.

Nefertiti was a perfect companion, especially as Jane's Parkinson's disease progressed. She was never underfoot, never jumped up onto the dining room table, and never broke anything. When she passed, we were devastated. It takes another pet owner to understand the emotion one experiences with the loss of a pet. A pet is a member of the family.

It takes a long time to get over the loss of a pet. Some people mitigate the loss by quickly obtaining a replacement.

We considered getting a kitten, or a pair of kittens, but dismissed the idea. At the time, we were traveling a lot and felt it would not be fair to an animal for us to be away for extended periods. We also now realize that having a kitten or a puppy tearing around the house would not have been advisable since Jane was experiencing serious mobility issues. The risk of falling might increase with a young animal in the house.

A few years ago, a longtime friend and professional associate of mine died from multiple causes. Let us call my friend "Roger." Part of the cause of death was bringing a young dog into his Roger's life when he was severely immunocompromised. It was a pet mismatch.

For many years, Roger had enjoyed the company of an Old English Sheepdog. Roger and his wife dearly loved the dog. So, when the dog died of old age, they immediately adopted an Old English Sheepdog puppy. I called the dog "energy with fur."

Roger's doctor warned him that he must avoid injury from the playful dog. In Florida, if a man wears long trousers, it is called "Florida formal," so most guys wear shorts most of the time. Roger was always in shorts! His doctor told him he must wear long trousers, blue jeans preferred, to avoid any skin tears from the dog's enthusiastic behavior. Roger refused to do so.

One day, the dog was so excited to see Roger come home from being out, that he jumped up on Roger, tearing the skin on his legs to shreds. The injury became infected. Roger was hospitalized. He died a few days later.

The message my friend Roger leaves is that one must match a pet to a person's health, and his or her stage in life. For someone with Parkinson's disease, a young dog or cat may add to the risk of fall and that fall might prove life altering or even fatal. A mature dog or cat might not provide the same risk. You must decide what works for you.

Suppose a PWP does want a dog to provide comfort and assistance. An assistance dog may be the answer.

If you would like to get an assistance dog, or have your dog trained for that job, contact: https://assistancedogsinternational.org/

Back to Jane and our pet story. Jane was devastated by the loss of our dear friend Nefertiti. Nefi passed early in the year. Valentine's Day was coming. I purchased a child's stuffed animal for Jane, a seal-point Siamese cat. She named it Nefi! After a few months, Jane felt Nefi needed a companion, so she purchased a white kitty which she named Muffin. A few years later, a third kitty arrived, this one a chocolate-point Siamese kitten, which I named Chocolate Drop.

The reader may wonder why we are telling you our stuffed animal story. The reason is that we have grown to love these little stuffed animals. Every time we look at them, we are reminded of the many wonderful creatures we have experienced in our lives. Our kitties may not be real, but they bring us pleasure. That is a good thing!

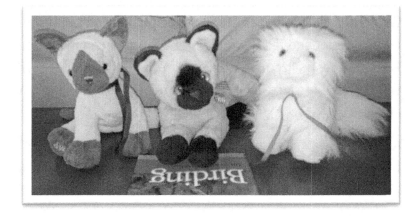

Chocolate Drop, Nefertiti, and Muffin Studying Jane's Cousin Kathern J. Schneider's Book, **Birding The Hudson Valley!**

Here is a book worth reading:

The Velveteen Rabbit (or How Toys Become Real) is a British children's book written by Margery Williams (also known as Margery Williams Bianco) and illustrated by William Nicholson. It chronicles the story of a stuffed rabbit's desire to become real through the love of his owner. The book was first published in 1922 and has been republished many times since.

Our message to you is that Parkinson's disease is going to change your life. Do not let it get you down. Adapt. If your friends feel you are a little weird by having a few stuffed animals in the house instead of "real" pets, so be it.

Our message goes well beyond Parkinson's and pets. Do what makes you happy. Singles and couples living with Parkinson's disease must accept change and adapt. Day-to-day living will change. Do not abandon intimacy; adapt. Do not sequester yourself in your home. Get out and mingle. Your circle of friends will change but friendship need not change. You can have a rewarding life while living with Parkinson's disease. We are proof of that!

APPENDIX

Abbreviations

DBS	Deep Brain Stimulator
MDVIP	Medical Doctors Versed in Prevention
PCP	Personal Care Physician
PD	Parkinson's Disease
PT	Physical Therapist
PWP	Person with Parkinson's disease
OT	Occupational Therapist
UTI	Urinary Tract Infection

Internet Links

Chapter 2 – Obtaining Great Medical Care

Medical Doctors Versed in Prevention (MDVIP)

https://www.mdvip.com/

Michael J. Fox Foundation for Parkinson's Research

https://www.michaeljfox.org/

Parkinson's Foundation

https://www.parkinson.org/

Centers of Excellence

https://www.parkinson.org/expert-care/centers-of-excellence

Chapter 3 – Learning from Others

Nextdoor

https://nextdoor.com/

Parkinson's Foundation

https://www.parkinson.org/

Michael J. Fox Foundation

https://www.michaeljfox.org/

Davis Phinney Foundation for Parkinson's
https://davisphinneyfoundation.org/

American Parkinson Disease Association

https://www.apdaparkinson.org/

Neuro Challenge Foundation for Parkinson's

https://www.neurochallenge.org/

Brain and Life Magazine

https://www.brainandlife.org/

The Great Courses

https://www.thegreatcourses.com/

Wondrium

https://www.wondrium.com/

Chapter 4 – Exercise

LSVT Big

https://www.lsvtglobal.com/LSVTBig

Rock Steady Boxing

https://rocksteadyboxing.org

General:

https://www.parkinson.org/pd-library/fact-sheets/Exercise-and-Parkinsons

Chapter 7 – How to Unfreeze

https://www.apdaparkinson.org/article/freezing-gait-and-parkinsons-disease/

https://parkinson.org/sites/default/files/Freezing-and-Parkinsons.pdf

Chapter 8 – Speaking Loudly and Clearly

Voice Aerobics

https://voiceaerobicsdvd.com/

Chapter 9 – Making the Home Parkinson's Friendly

ADA Compliance

https://www.ada-compliance.com/ada-compliance/ada-ramp

Chapter 14 – Urinary Incontinence

PureWick

https://www.purewickathome.com/

Chapter 16 — Do not Fall—Use an Assist Device

U-Step walker

https://www.ustep.com/

Chapter 17 – Increasing Your Mobility

TravelScoot scooter

https://www.travelscootusa.com

Chapter 19 – Off to the Hospital

https://www.parkinson.org/Living-with-Parkinsons/Resources-and-Support/Hospital-Kit

Chapter 20 - Where to Go if You Need Rehabilitation

American Hospital Association

https://www.aha.org/

Chapter 22 – Flying

Federal Aviation Administration

https://www.faa.gov/

Chapter 24 – Parkinson's and Pets

Assistance Dogs International

https://assistancedogsinternational.org/

Books

Parkinson's Treatment - 10 Secrets to a Happier Life, Michael S. Okun, M.D.

10 Breakthrough Therapies for Parkinson's Disease, Michael S. Okun, M.D.

Ask the Doctor about Parkinson's Disease, Michael S. Okun, M.D., Hubert H. Fernandez, M.D.

Living with Parkinson's Disease – A Complete Guide for Patients and Caregivers, Michael S. Okun, M.D., Irene A. Malaty, M.D., Wissam Debb, M.D.

The Muhammad Ali Parkinson Center 100 Question and Answers about Parkinson's Disease, Abraham Lieberman, M.D.

Every Victory Counts, Davis Phinney Foundation, Monique Giroux, M.D., Sierra Farris, PA-C, IPAS, plus 40 other contributors. Order directly from the Foundation.

300 Tips for Making Life Easier, Parkinson's Disease, Second Edition, Shelly Peterman Schwarz

RECOGNITION

There are many people to thank for making this book happen.

We have given our presentation "Ideas for Living Well with Parkinson's Disease" to hundreds of people over a five year period. Some suggested we write a book so that our experience could be available to more people. We listened, and finally acted. We did not keep a record of who made a recommendation. Although unnamed, our thanks go out to them.

Without our resolute editors, this book would not have published. A special thanks to the following:

Elizabeth Costello, Jane's life-long friend and English language professional, for her meticulous proofreading/copyediting.

Cynthia Gay, a dedicated Parkinson's disease caregiver, and English language college graduate, for her skilled editing.

Fred and Pat Purello who did a final review, checking every word and every punctuation mark.

Connie and Matt Maher for volunteering to be the couple on the bench on the book's front cover, and for their review of content.

Don Landy, our friend, former neighbor, and author, for his encouragement for us to speak from the heart as we tell our story of living with Parkinson's disease.

We are indebted to those who took the time to review our writings, critique them for content, and make suggestions. Thanks go out to Dawn S. Shore, Cheryl S. Dean, Elizabeth Straitiff, and Carolyn McDermott.

Made in United States
Orlando, FL
19 April 2022

17007392R20063